Deadly Biocultures

An earlier version of chapter 1 was published as Nadine Ehlers and Shiloh Krupar, "Hope Logics: Biomedicine, Affective Conventions of Cancer, and the Governing of Biocitizenry," *Configurations* 23, no. 1 (2015): 385–413; copyright 2014 by The Johns Hopkins University Press. A different version of chapter 2 was published as Shiloh Krupar and Nadine Ehlers, "Target: Biomedicine and Racialized Geo-body-politics," *Occasion* 8 (2015), https://arcade.stanford.edu/occasion/target-biomedicine-and -racialized-geo-body-politics; made available to the public by a Creative Commons Attribution-NonCommercial-ShareAlike 3.0 United States License. Chapter 2, in modified form, was published as Shiloh Krupar and Nadine Ehlers, "Biofutures: Race and the Governance of Health," *Environment and Planning D: Society and Space* 35, no. 2 (2017): 222–40; reprinted by permission of SAGE Publications, Ltd.; http:// journals.sagepub.com/doi/abs/10.1177/0263775816654475. A different version of chapter 4 was published as Nadine Ehlers, "Fat Is the Future: Bioprospecting, Fat Stem Cells, and Emergent Breasted Materialities," in *Fat: Culture and Materiality,* ed. Christopher Forth and Alison Leitch (London: Bloomsbury, 2014), 109–22; reprinted by permission of Bloomsbury Academic, imprint of Bloomsbury Publishing Plc. Parts of chapter 5 were published as Shiloh Krupar, "Green Death: Sustainability and the Administration of the Dead," *cultural geographies* 25, no. 2 (2018): 267–84; reprinted by permission of SAGE Publications, Ltd.; http://journals.sagepub.com/doi /abs/10.1177/1474474017732977.

Published by the University of Minnesota Press
111 Third Avenue South, Suite 290
Minneapolis, MN 55401-2520
http://www.upress.umn.edu

ISBN 978-1-5179-0506-4 (hc)
ISBN 978-1-5179-0507-1 (pb)

A Cataloging-in-Publication record is available from the Library of Congress.

Printed in the United States of America on acid-free paper

The University of Minnesota is an equal-opportunity educator and employer.

Curiosity . . . the word . . . evokes "concern"; it evokes the
care one takes for what exists and could exist; a readiness
to find strange and singular what surrounds us; a certain
relentlessness to break up our familiarities and to regard
otherwise the same things; a fervor to grasp what is happening
and what passes; a casualness in regard to the traditional
hierarchies of the important and the essential. I dream of a
new age of curiosity.

—MICHEL FOUCAULT, "THE MASKED PHILOSOPHER"

Contents

Acknowledgments

The research for this book began many years ago, and the project has taken various forms rooted in different locations and communities. As such, more people made this work possible than we have room to list. Jason Weidemann welcomed this book at the University of Minnesota Press, and we would like to thank him for his support and conviction about the project. The insights of two anonymous reviewers helped crystallize our thinking, and we appreciate their intellectual generosity. Shiloh Krupar is grateful for the ongoing camaraderie, unassailable humor, and inspirational work of C. Greig Crysler, Sarah Kanouse, Jenna Loyd, Kate Chandler, Jason Moore and Diana Gildea, Rebecca Lave, the Administration, and Michele Pred. At Georgetown University, she thanks the intellectual capaciousness of the Culture and Politics program and its incredible students and network of CULP-minded colleagues. Nadine Ehlers could not ask for a better set of colleagues at the University of Sydney. In particular, Melinda Cooper, Dinesh Wadiwel, Sonja Van Wichelen, and Rebecca Scott Bray have been formidable interlocutors and offered an amazingly supportive environment.

Each of the chapters here owes a debt of thanks to a range of individuals. In relation to our work on hope, Bob Carey continues to be a major inspiration. Our research on targeting has benefited from the opportunities and insights shared by Wendy Cheng, Rashad Shabazz, Sara H. Smith, Pavithra Vasudevan, and Laura Liu. We are thankful to Melinda Cooper and Cathy Waldby for advancing our thinking about the affirmation to thrive and for sage advice about the book as a whole. Finally, research on greening the afterlife was supported by *cultural geographies* editor Dydia DeLyser, Dinesh Wadiwel, the research assistance of Ivy Otradovec, and the staff at the Congressional Cemetery in Washington, D.C., and at Anderson McQueen Funeral Home in St. Petersburg, Florida.

We're grateful for the opportunities we've had to present parts of our research collaboratively and individually at conferences, including the American Studies Association and the American Association of Geographers, and an intensive—and incredibly generative—book forum hosted by the Biopolitics of Science Research Network at the University of Sydney in 2017.

The research for this book was supported by a number of small grants. At Georgetown, Shiloh was the recipient of several School of Foreign Service semester-based and summer grants that enabled her progress on the book; the FSF MAPWISELY grant funded her travel for the book workshop in Sydney. At the University of Sydney, Nadine was supported by the Faculty of Arts and Social Sciences Research Support Scheme, the School of Social and Political Sciences Conference Funding Scheme, and various other avenues of research assistance.

On a personal note, Nadine would like to thank Shiloh more than anyone. This work—and the various forms it has taken over the years—has been possible only because of an initial serendipity involving an orange dress. Cowriter, co-conspirator, and fierce friend, Shiloh has pushed my thinking in directions I didn't know existed. To Duncan, Imogen, and Maiya Ehlers, my indomitable grandmother, Domna Daciw, and to Kirsty and Phoebe Nowlan, Clare Armitage, Arabella Hayes, Donette Francis, and Leslie Hinkson, thank you for being my anchors.

Shiloh sends her deepest gratitude to Nadine: our intellectual companionship and friendship have made (academic) life inhabitable when it is not and galvanized an uncompromising interdisciplinarity and commitment to critique that will endure through my lifetime. Special thanks also to Joshua McDonald for his infectious wit, intellect, musical fraternizing, and editorial skills; the National Toxic Land/Labor Conservation Service; Calamity Row; D.C. geographers; Wendy Morrison; Chris Lehmann; Joe McGill and Astra Rooney; Harlan, Francis, Grummitch, and Harriet; the late Allan Pred; Jason and Carmen Krupar; and my parents, Joseph and Karen Krupar, for their inexhaustible generosity, dynamic minds, and delight in the absurd.

When the book is at its best, it is because of this generous support network. Any errors or misunderstandings in this volume are ours alone.

Introduction

Biocultures

Life-making occupies the biomedical imaginary in late Western liberalism.[1] Life-making encapsulates all those contemporary efforts to make people live *more*—to exponentially expand their capacities for life, to optimize and extend what counts as life, and to encourage people to pursue positive life-enhancing practices. This quest for more life can be seen across a range of activities, practices, and technologies that compose what we name *biocultures* in the United States: those cultural spheres where biomedicine extends beyond the formal institutions of the clinic, the hospital, the lab, and so forth and is incorporated into broader social practices and rationalities. Biocultures foreground the pursuit of life and are linked to contemporary biomedicine and public health, operating at the individual, collective, and institutional levels. Biocultures are enmeshed with the biomedical pursuit of fostering biological life—understanding, treating, and preventing disease—and, within biocultures, life is increasingly viewed through the lens of biomedical logics, innovations, and possibilities.

Biocultures thus highlight how biomedicine has become central to everyday life—our relationships to self and to others. For instance, we now track our steps, sleep patterns, and caloric intake. We survey and monitor ourselves for the smallest signs of illness or bodily anomaly. We anticipate potential futures of disease and take on broader health directives as personal pursuits. We share and compare our health status, and this status has become a key mode through which we understand ourselves and our relationships. As Nikolas Rose has stated, "biomedicine . . . has thus not simply changed our relation to health and illness but has modified the things we think we might hope for and the objectives we aspire to. That is to say, it has helped make us the kinds of people we have become."[2] These everyday understandings and experiences of health are shaped by the broader *biomedicalization* of the U.S. social landscape, where almost anything now is cast as a biomedical problem.[3] According to Adele Clarke et al., biomedicalization involves a heightened focus on risk and

1

surveillance, the increasingly technoscientific nature of biomedical practices and innovations, the privatization and corporatization of biomedicine,
and the increase in production and transmission of health/medical knowledges across multiple arenas of society.[4]

The life-making pursuit within biocultures seems like a profoundly positive venture. However, this book insists that life-making is inseparable from
relations of power. While life-making clearly affirms life, this affirmation
of life—and the effort to make people live more—is regulatory. In other
words, life-making operates as a *regulatory politics of affirmation*.[5] Life-
making governs by orienting people toward certain ways of looking after
themselves, particular goals of health, and constrained understandings of
body and self.

To examine the governing functions and regulatory nature of life-
making, we draw on the work of Michel Foucault. Foucault uses the concept
of *government* broadly to encapsulate various ways that humans are guided:
rather than being restricted to management by the state or an administration, government also addresses "problems of self-control, guidance for the
family and for children, management of the household, directing the soul,
and other questions."[6] Foucault deploys the term *life* to refer to the conditioning of biological capacities of the individual and the population and
how these capacities are inextricable from the logics of governing. Foucault
does not propose an ontology of life; rather, his concern is how biological
life comes to be known and conditioned through various mechanisms
and techniques—power/knowledge relations—that constitute a specific
modern form of power Foucault named *biopower.* Within biopower, "life"
emerges as central to political strategies: biopower operates "to incite, re-
inforce, control, monitor, optimize, and organize the forces under it: [it
is] a power bent on generating forces, making them grow, and ordering
them, rather than one dedicated to impeding them, making them submit,
or destroying them."[7] This biopower, as Foucault tells us, has assumed two
basic forms.

One form, which Foucault called *biopolitics,* focuses on the level of the
population. It is "the series of governmental strategies centered on this new
concept called 'life.'"[8] Biopolitics thus marks the historical rise of biological
life as the object of state calculation and strategy, which takes "the total-
ity of the concrete processes of life in a population . . . [as] the target of . . .
security."[9] This modern and productive form of power historically entailed
establishing regulatory controls over a range of biological processes (birth,

mortality, disease incidence, and so forth) so as to regularize the population, curtail unpredictability (in terms of disease, disasters, epidemics, etc.),
and achieve stability across the population. Biopolitics, then, refers to the
series of techniques, technologies, relays, and operations that, in Foucault's
intriguing words, *"make live."*[10] In its most basic formulation, the function
to "make live" within biopolitical operations concerns the managing and
fostering of life in its generality. It is the calculated management of life that
engenders and develops life in certain directions to produce and enhance
capacities: "to improve life, to prolong its duration, to improve its chances,
to avoid accidents, and to compensate for [its] failings."[11]

The second form of biopower, which Foucault called *discipline* (or, alter-
natively, the anatamo-politics of the human body), operates inside institutions, focuses on individual bodies, and takes the individual body as a target
to produce a docile, useful, productive subject.[12] Discipline refers to that set
of practices that endows the individual body with capacities and "'makes'
individuals; it is the specific technique of a power that regards individuals
both as objects and as instruments of its exercise."[13] Individuals are both
the target of disciplinary power and its vehicles, in that they reproduce it
through incorporating discipline into their formation of self. This body
that is individualized, and the individual that is made, emerge in relation to
sets of norms and normalizing technologies. In this emergence, the subject
actively participates in forming the self in line with norms.[14]

Biopolitics uses, infiltrates, and embeds itself into disciplinary techniques[15]—obliging individuals to enter themselves into the discourses of
"life" so that they can then be advised how—through discipline—to lead
a life, conduct themselves, and care for the self.[16] The "ends" of this form
of biological governing concern the control, stabilizing, and improvement
of life. In other words, to "make live" becomes a biopolitical—and then
often disciplinary—imperative.[17] The individual is reworked with respect
to the population for certain normalizing (and standardizing) ends, as a
living being that is prosperous and productive for society.[18] Conversely,
subjects become invested—entering themselves to this governing function
of biopolitics—"if ... [they] want to be protected, assisted, taken charge
of—if, in other words, ... [they] want happiness and well-being. ... The
state of prosperity will be the rallying cry of all the discourses and practices
affiliated to this form of power."[19] Biopolitical "make live" logics are thus
transposed into various forms of discipline.

In short, biopolitics affirms life through the imperative to "make live" and can thus be said to be a politics of affirmation. It orients the biological—living beings—*toward life* in a regulatory fashion. As such, this affirmation cannot be seen as neutral or liberatory; it is not necessarily "good." Rather, it is crucial we recognize that life can only exist under certain conditions; it is contoured in particular ways; and some ways of living, not to mention forms of life, are valued above others. Foucault famously referred to the stratification of life-making in terms of a "make live/let die" relationship.[20] Life-making is "known" and configured as ontologically good because affirming life has traditionally operated to protect the population from risk, to guide the health of individuals toward a standardized norm, and to foster the lives of the individuals who comprise the nation. However, the twin operation of *let die* reveals that such life-making actually augments social disparities and, in its extreme, kills. Not all forms of life are fostered equally; indeed, the life possibilities of some are produced through limiting the lives of others. According to Foucault, "letting die" is integral to the biopolitical imperative to "make live" and entails various operations of abandonment, negligence, and oversight: "in modernity, making live and letting die become logical correlates."[21] Owing to the vicissitudes of resource allocation and social stratification, some are made to live (more) at the expense of others.[22] There are clear disparities in the possibilities for health and life produced through the structural and ideological workings of race, class, sexuality, gender, and other geopolitical and geographical specificities. Such inequities in the ability to pursue life or to have one's life affirmed have been theorized in a range of ways—as social death, premature death, slow death, and—as we argue in this book—*deadly life-making*.[23]

This book uses the phrase *deadly life-making* to examine the centrality of "letting die" to "making live" and the unequal enhancement of life under biopolitics; it insists that we recognize death is always inside life and inextricable from processes of life-making. Three forms of "letting die" shape the terrain of the contemporary U.S. biocultures that we analyze throughout this volume: these are not discrete but mutually condition one another.[24] First, life-making practices can *obscure death*: the very processes that affirm life can invisibilize the deaths that continue to occur despite efforts to make live; or, due to the focus on enhancing the lives of one part of the population, other segments of the population and their limited life chances are ignored. Additionally, those who live in the folds of death—vulnerable individuals or those facing imminent death—are often overlooked. Second, life-making practices can *create deathly conditions* (that might also be obscured), such as reproducing inequities in prevention, access to health services, and treatment—at policy, political economy, and institutional levels; addressing risk as a bodily property rather than as socially produced, thus allowing the causes to continue; and designating certain individuals and communities as higher risk and/or risky and therefore in need of separation, leading to inadequate or rationed care. Third, efforts to "make live" can *produce death and/or death effects*: the very operations that are ostensibly said to make people live can kill; certain individuals and communities are subject to even more precarity, leading to exponential deaths of some over others; taking a predominately biomedical approach to health obscures the political economy of health, which, in turn, precipitates more deaths. Importantly, our understanding of death here is informed by Foucault's dictum: "when I say 'killing,' I obviously do not mean simply murder as such, but also every form of indirect murder: the fact of exposing someone to death, increasing the risk of death for some people, or, quite simply, political death, expulsion, rejection, and so on."[25]

We look at these death-in-life dimensions in U.S. biocultures specifically in the context of what Melinda Cooper names "neoliberal biopolitics."[26] For our purposes, *neoliberal biopolitics* functions within the broader historical terrain of late liberalism and may be characterized by the following logics and practices: a declining welfare imperative, the increasing absence of the idea of society or of a collective social good, and a heightened individualizing of the administration and management of life and risk (in contradistinction to an earlier regularizing of life and collectivizing of risk). In this context, biopolitical operations continue to structure the politics of life in the United States, but often with specifically neoliberal rationalities and policies. While people are called on to participate in life-making as if it were unquestionably good, the operations of "make live" are attenuated and/or redirected: neoliberal biopolitics fosters health and life in relation to market logics, intensifies speculation in ways that gamble with life-and-death stakes of biological existence, and places the onus for health on the individual. The individual now is positioned as solely responsible for being healthy and maintaining health, and those who fail to "live properly" are often not supported and/or denigrated.

Moreover, rather than standardizing, normalizing, and protecting the life of the population, neoliberal life-making, in the context of biomedicine, customizes biological life—reworking it beyond its perceived limits—and, more broadly, capitalizes on the life opportunities of diverse populations and individuals. Such operations can be linked to changes in biomedicine itself. In contradistinction to an earlier welfare-oriented health arena, the latter half of the twentieth century—what is called the neoliberal era—has seen a modification and transformation of biomedicine: there is an increased focus on customizing the body rather than normalizing; there has been a rise of an all-encompassing and pervasive regime of "health"; and life has been geneticized and molecularized, leading to expanding opportunities to further individualize life and intimately govern everyday life. Moreover, we see an intensification of efforts to generate value through processes of both "making live" and "letting die"—particularly in relation to the corporatization of health care and biomedicine. Rather than warding off risk, precarity and the contingencies of life and death become opportunities for financial gain, cost–benefit efficiencies, heightened individual and group administration, and the hierarchical ordering of social groups. In short, under neoliberal biopolitics, health care and biomedical technologies are increasingly financialized and customized in ways that risk further stratifying life based on race, class, gender, disability, and so on.

This book foregrounds how these specificities of neoliberal biopolitics—particularly as they relate to biomedicine—contour both life-making practices and processes of letting die in key biocultures of the United States. We focus on the United States precisely because of the prominent ways that neoliberal rationalities and policies operate in/through biomedicine and health care provision in this arena—which models effects that are present or developing in other national contexts to varying degrees. Moreover, we are interested in life-making as a mode of governing in the United States because of the complex ways that "affirmation" works in the American context, which contradictorily advocates "freedom" and "happiness" as cultural goals within a larger endorsement of competition, scarcity, deservingness, and violence. In other words, U.S. neoliberal biopolitics imbricates make live/let die in complex ways that exacerbate inequalities and exclusions under liberalism. Finally, the diversity of U.S. biocultures reveals complex convergences of culture and biomedicine that scholars and students may find instructive when investigating non-American biocultural arenas—that is, potentially similar to and/or influenced by the United States in the geopolitics of global health policy and wider developments of biocitizenship on local to international scales.[27]

Our analysis features *biocultures* as an arena and methodology. Biocultures address a particular health issue terrain, and each is delimited by a set of knowledges as they are bound up in specific practices and relations of power. Each bioculture we examine here is structured through *a central affirmation—an ostensibly positive "truth claim"*—that regulates and intimately governs that sphere. That affirmation organizes the social in relation to that particular sphere (i.e., individuals, goods and services, infrastructures, etc.) and the biological materiality of the body that is the object of that sphere. Affirmations guide and discipline individuals, communities, and polities in relation to a particular biomedically framed problem or issue; each affirmation we look at affirms life, yet does so in a constrained way (precisely because it is a truth claim—a limited way of understanding something). Thus we look at the deathly dimensions of these affirmations as they operate in specific biocultural arenas: those related to cancer, racial health, obesity, stem cells, aging, and corpse disposal.

Biocultures are composed of numerous actors—the "subjects" of the bioculture—such as clinicians, policy makers, health care providers and industry partners, media and advertisers, social organizations and community actors, activists, artists, and other individuals. Biocultures operate across scales, from the individual biomedical subject or consumer to broader biomedical logics and governance. Within biocultures, specific technologies and techniques—that is, clinical directives and protocols, policy goals, economic formulas and tools—are deployed to speak about the subject or self of the particular bioculture and to structure/govern its existence, giving rise to counter-truth claims that contest these dominant technologies and techniques. In looking at biocultures, this book prioritizes an intertextual reading between various kinds of cultural products, knowledges, practices, and "the real." Our readings cross scales of analysis and spaces of investigation—from the cellular to the body, the clinic, and national public policy—because the affirmations that we examine traverse and govern these sites. In doing so, we refuse a distinction between the "bio" and the "cultural," instead highlighting that the body and culture are never separate and that the biomedical arena and cultural practices are linked and mutually influential.[28] As we note further in this introduction, *Deadly Biocultures* engages with the growing literature on biocitizenship, biosociality, bioeconomy, biovalue, and biofutures; our focus on biocultures—their affirmation of life and attendant deathly effects—both draws on and contributes to these already circulating conversations that analyze ways of being and new regimes of governing through the lens of *bio*. The *bio*-prefix simultaneously refers to the biological material body and the ways this materiality is inextricable from broader political economic relations and social transformations.

In the chapters that follow, we consider the deathly conditions of contemporary life-making through investigating five key affirmations that circulate in particular U.S. biocultures: the affirmation to *hope,* the affirmation to *target,* the affirmation to *thrive,* the affirmation to *secure,* and the affirmation to *green.* Each individual chapter of this book takes a particular life/ death arena as its point of analysis and charts how that sphere is contoured and governed—in terms of neoliberal biopolitics and discipline—via one of these particular overarching affirmations. We demonstrate that the affirmation at work in these biocultures simultaneously affirms life and produces deathly conditions or death itself—to limit, curtail, forestall, or inhibit life. Given the imbrication of death-in-life—specifically in life-making practices and techniques—the five chapters call for a politics that is attentive to death, wherein death and forms of death-in-life are recognized as both the product of life-making practices and rhetoric and a potential social platform from which to affirm a different ethics or way of living. Coupled with the analysis of deadly life-making, then, each chapter also considers a politics or ethics that would be more attentive to the way life is disproportionately arranged and questions who is being "let die" and on what terms. Each chapter proposes how to activate that recognition of death-in-life as a vehicle for social change. This includes what we call *alternative biocultures/biofutures*—other ways that race, class, gender, age, sexuality, and disability might be mapped onto or intersect with biomedicine—and resistant individual practices and social forms that range from what might be thought of as abolitionist biomedicine to performances of irreverent vulnerability.

Chapter 1 explores how the affirmation of hope is used to orient individuals and the population more broadly toward vigilant survival following cancer diagnosis—to persist and affirm life through the individual and collective deployment of hope. Specifically, we argue that hope is framed as the principle affective means through which to fight cancer. Our central claim is that such fighting through hope, as seen in the endless pursuit of the biomedical cure and the "war on cancer," is never simply benign. Instead, dominant affective conventions of hope—that is, the perceptual, emotional, and corporeal modes of managing and responding to events—perform an intimate governing function within biocultures, at the scale of both biopolitical management and individual discipline. We argue that hope conditions (disciplines and regularizes) responses to bodily vulnerability and uncertainty and affirms life in ways that reproduce dominant bodily norms and that exclude or preclude the acknowledgment of vulnerability and the reality of death.

We ground these claims in an investigation of cancer activism and treatment and mark the ways the affirmation of hope has shifted from earlier national protection efforts to an individualized/biologized disposition and activity—specifically in relation to breast cancer. We show that in late liberalism, hope has become simultaneously commercialized mass spectacle and an optimistic—and at times militant—enterprise. The chapter details how hope is actively made and maintained within cancer-related biocultures—via what we call spectacles of hope, infrastructures of care, and bioethics of faith. Through case studies of practices and enactments of hope—from hospital architectural aesthetics to cancer-simulated video gameplay—we show that individuals who do not (or are not able to) embody dominant modes of hope, and thus fight cancer in a way that resounds in popular discourse, are framed as failed or negligent and invisibilized or abandoned within the cultural realm. Moreover, the insistence on hoping for the biomedical cure precludes a social justice approach that would actually apprehend the environmental, class-based, and racialized causes of cancer incidence and deaths. The chapter concludes by considering how individuals find other ways to live with and die from cancer, not through forsaking hope but through developing and practicing alternative hope tactics—"hoping for other things"—in relation to cancer.

Chapter 2 addresses the affirmation to target within the context of race-based health. Target technologies are ostensibly deployed to affirm life: they are said to enable the tailoring of biomedical attention and are advocated as the means through which to biopolitically foster the health of particular populations. While the chapter highlights the history of race-specific governing of health, we focus on two contemporary target technologies: the first race-based pharmaceutical—BiDil—approved by the U.S. Federal Drug Administration in 2005 and marketed as a drug specifically for self-identified black subjects that suffer from heart failure, and medical hot-spotting, a practice that began in Camden, New Jersey, in 2007 and that uses GIS technologies and spatial profiling to identify populations that are using health care resources at exorbitant rates (i.e., "super-users") to facilitate preemptive care. We argue that, despite efforts to ameliorate health disparities, targeting further subjects racial minorities—and specifically black subjects—to enduring inequities/iniquities and the cost–benefit logics of the U.S. health care system.[29]

We examine this argument across two scales: the administrative bio-political level, where racialized bodies are demarcated in space as targets requiring biomedical intervention, and the embodied level, where individual bodies and communities are disciplined through these technologies to racially target themselves and to embody race as a biological ontology. Our central claim is that race-specific pharmaceuticals and medical hot-spotting position race as a proxy for corporeal/genetic truth, geopolitically delimit life, and threaten to make health and other social inequalities even worse. In the case of BiDil, race is ontologized as/for a market; accumulation is achieved through customization. Medical hot-spotting, by contrast, ontologizes race in/as space to secure cost efficiencies in the U.S. health care system and minimize uncompensated-care debt. While these target technologies are said to promote the life of vulnerable populations, they also limit how that life can be lived—whether through logics of spatial apartheid or of structural abandonment. What is called for is an "abolitionist biomedicine" that recognizes and seeks to challenge the multifarious ways that race is ontologized as a corporeal and/or spatial truth while attending to the very real embodied effects of structural racism.

Chapter 3 analyzes the affirmation to thrive in relation to fatness/fat and the accompanying "economy of fat" in two biocultural domains. First, we look at biomedical and public health practices that work to eradicate fat from the body—wherein obesity is framed as resulting in an individual's "failure to thrive." Various neoliberal biopolitical and disciplinary techniques—from healthy school lunches to fitness campaigns and surgical interventions (gastric banding, bypass, or sleeve surgeries)—are lauded as both reducing surplus fat and helping people to thrive: to live more. As we show, however, biomedical and public health approaches can simultaneously advance and compromise obesity reduction. They generally fail to address the structural conditions that produce obesity and make it an "unequal opportunity disease." Furthermore, in not addressing structural conditions, these approaches can sustain (and are at times complicit in) the prevalence of obesity and industry/private-sector exploitation of fatness—where the fat body is commodified as a source of value with infinite cash-generating potential, whether through the fast-food or the diet and fitness industry.

Second, we examine the rise of fat harvesting in regenerative medicine. In this domain, fat (adipose tissue) is harnessed and instrumentalized as a form of biovalue that can generate more life, precisely because it has been identified as a rich source of multipotent stem cells that can be directed to grow into bone, cartilage, and tissue. As such, fat promises to become the "gold standard" in corporeal repair and is being cryopreserved (in the form of fat banking) in anticipation of future applications. Yet, while the thriving of fat—through stem cell proliferation—represents a new horizon in the biomedical fostering of life, only those already privileged within circuits of capital can access these technologies. Moreover, cells might proliferate too well, and their excessive vitality might result in the material emergence of cancer. The fat cell, as we see, is differently valued according to the body in which it is located. Furthermore, it at once represents the impediment to and means through which to thrive, and in both domains, fat kills or is said to kill—but offers the material ground for exploitation. We explore what ethical avenues might be available for recognizing the death effects of the affirmation to thrive and call for more inclusive and socially accountable ways to thrive.

Chapter 4 explores the affirmation to secure the life of the aging subject and to secure *against* aging and decline. In biocultures of aging, to "secure" refers to safeguarding individuals against the ravages of old age. But aging and old age have long been associated with dependency, pathology, and declining productivity and are tethered to ideas of fiscal burden and national decay. Aging therefore functions as a broader security problematic for biopolitics, inspiring strategies that enhance the population and the individual's capacity to live more and age successfully, and that separate out bodies in decline and secure against the costs of dependent aging populations.

The first part of the chapter examines efforts to secure "aging well." On one hand, this entails the interrelated promotion of longevity, independent living, and functional aging that ostensibly enable individuals to maximize "third age"—a life-phase/stage in which older individuals are able to partake in an active, personally fulfilling, healthy life after the constraints of work and child-rearing. On the other hand, we observe the biofinancialization of old age: reducing life to a funding problem through economic thinking to assess the burden of "age-related decline" and preempt the cost of age-impaired states of the population. While by no means an exhaustive account of the dynamic biocultural arena of aging, these cases map how the affirmation to secure "aging well" supports and organizes particular kinds of aging and life maintenance; we highlight the social costs of promoting third age and ways that biofinancializing old age may discount and imperil certain lives.

For the second part of the chapter, we consider forms of "governing decline" that stretch into the very last moments of life and structure expectations of "what should be done" for and to the elderly. We examine two key areas of the governing of age-related decline: first, the relentless biomedical efforts to extend the lives of ailing older individuals—the logic of "more life at any cost" and its limitations—and second, the economic rationalities that condition the treatment of older individuals and the regimes of care in the extrabiomedical environments of nursing homes and hospice care. We argue that rather than securing the lives of those on the event horizon of life, these extrabiomedical sites can be considered "shadowlands," where those in deep old age are subject to forms of "deadly care" and often abandoned. Concluding the chapter, we ask, what alternative biocultures of aging might exist or be imagined to reaffirm aging based on more positive understandings of dependency in older age and vulnerability as integral to life and social relationships?

Our final chapter shifts to the neoliberal biopolitical relations of life-making and "letting die" in what may seem at first an unlikely biocultural arena: the afterlife of the dead human body. Chapter 5 thus moves more fully into extrabiomedical spheres to critically survey contemporary disposal technologies and commemorative efforts that seek to "green" the dead human body, from recycling body parts to returning the corpse to nature. These practices—operating under what we see as the affirmation to green—*extend* the biomedical truth discourse of affirming life by affirming the "afterlife": as an opportunity to generate new markets and efficiencies through bioremediation of the body and through the production of legacy for some. The body after death offers an expanded field of material possibilities to convert corporeality into forms of value. In one instance, the body/parts are converted into financial value, and in the other, the corpse becomes a material input for nature and a vehicle for legacy/commemoration that validates the value of a life lived. For our first empirical case, we observe efforts to create new efficiencies in corpse disposal and new markets centered on the material vitality of the dead body. For example, we look at carbon-neutral cremation, orthopedic implant recycling, and body expungement following medical donation/scientific gift. Together, these practices exemplify the pursuit of "no remains" within late liberal biocultures. For the second case, we look at a range of examples—from green burial to eternal reefs and transgenic tombstones—that endeavor to redeem the dead body's decomposition as natural and reimagine/resituate the body as part of the natural world.

Bioremediation ostensibly demonstrates an ethical and/or economic commitment to affirming the greening of afterlife. At the same time, valuing bioremediation on the basis of greening actually obscures a long history and present application of bioremediation of minorities, women, the mentally ill, the poor/indigent (for instance, the experimentation on racial minorities, biopiracy, the contemporary clinical labor of nonwhite and non-Western subjects). Efforts to put the dead body to work in new ways risk orchestrating efficiencies that legitimate a predatory death industry and the status quo characterized by excessive consumption. Moreover, in the case of greening the disposal of one's body as a gift to nature and/or sustainable legacy, the underside of this bioremediation is that it further entrenches social position in life: only those privileged in life have control over their own human remains and material traces after death. It is also an act haunted by a legacy of mass disappearance, disposability, and violent human–nonhuman and person–thing social divisions. In response to these practices, we explore an environmental ethics of human remains that contributes to rather than eclipses environmental justice and civil rights projects.

The book's coda considers the overarching effects of insistent life-making and how we might pursue creative ways to resist/re-work the intimate governing operations of affirmation. We elaborate on what a politics attentive to death might mean and meditate on possible avenues for "living on"—enduring—in the context of deadly life-making.

Throughout these chapters, *Deadly Biocultures* is in conversation with a rich field of research literature on biomedicine and the integration of the biological body with social, political, and economic relations. As we noted earlier, such research corresponds with what has been a proliferation of conceptual frameworks tied to vocabulary with the *bio-* prefix in recent decades. For example, Nikolas Rose and Carlos Novas deploy the term *biocitizenship* to describe an active form of citizenship that has emerged in late liberalism, one that produces new forms of belonging, claims to knowledge and expertise, and access to resources predicated on biological factors.[30] Paul Rabinow proposed the concept of *biosociality* to mark how individuals have now formed social relationships and produced collective notions of identity based on shared genetic or biological conditions.[31]

Catherine Waldby developed the term *biovalue* to explain "the yield of vitality produced by the biotechnical reformulation of living processes."[32] She focuses specifically on how biotechnology intervenes between certain living and nonliving systems such that "new and contingent forms of vitality can be created, capitalizing on life."[33] Rose later uses the term somewhat differently, to refer to "the value to be extracted from the vital properties of living processes."[34] Alongside the notion of biovalue, Kaushik Sunder Rajan and Melinda Cooper have independently explored the concept of *biocapital* and enriched our understandings of the imbrications of biology with contemporary conceptions of life and life-forms.[35] The proliferation and uptake of these terms indicate the critical importance of understanding the operations of biomedicine and biological materials and new modes of being, socializing, valuing, and governing within society and politics. Each of these terms is a practical tool of thought supported by discipline-specific methods and empirical work as well as cross-disciplinary and cross-professional conversations and research.

Deadly Biocultures moves within these critical traditions to take a broad approach to analyzing the biomedicalization of life. At the same time, it offers a methodology that is distinct from other important accounts of emerging regimes of governing biological life. As we previously described, the book investigates what we call *biocultures* in late liberalism. This allows us to take an expansive view to the ways life-making operates through linkages between biomedical protocols and practices, social movements, cultural norms around health, and individual choices.[36] Our interest in biocultures as a methodology seeks to widen the analysis of neoliberalism and biopolitics beyond a topical concentration on biotech and biomedicine; our aim is to provide a critical tool to examine how biomedical rationalities extend across scales and circulate in wider cultural domains within the United States.

This book is also aligned with contemporary theory and scholarship that addresses the politics of life and death. We draw on empirical case materials that span public policy and campaigns, to drug-sponsored advertisements and video games, to apprehend the messy entanglements of life and death. Our approach focuses on contemporary efforts of life-*making* that are bound up with forms of death. A number of biopolitical theorists have been attentive to the presence and operations of death in the politics of life. Roberto Esposito, for instance, has argued that biopolitics is characterized by an inherent thanatopolitical logic. Death, according to Esposito, is a structural necessity in the advancement of life, and the protection of life necessarily reverses into the production of death: the advancement of life and its elimination are opposing dimensions in Esposito's view, and defense and death are key features of modern politics.[37] Giorgio Agamben likewise centralizes death in his understanding of biopolitics. He proposes that the politics of life is predicated on a binary or distinction between *zoe* (bare human life reduced to merely being alive) and *bios* (the life of humans as rights bearing/as lives worth living). Importantly, for Agamben, *bios* can be reduced to *zoe* (where life is abandoned and exposed to death) through operations of sovereign power in states of exception.[38] Additionally, Achille Mbembe has provocatively advanced the notion of "necropolitics" to describe the enactment of sovereignty in cases where "the generalized instrumentalization of human existence and the material destruction of human bodies and populations" are the central project of power.[39]

While acknowledging that sovereign power (as an absolute form of dominating power) may become established (and exercised) through a political order focused on life, this book refuses the idea that life and death are binary or oppositional or that death is exceptional. Instead, it explores how *death is folded into life through intimate and often mundane forms of governing.* Distinct from efforts to theorize life or death as an ontology and state of being, our methodological attention to biomedical rationalities and modes of governance accounts for the ways different practices of life-making and affirmations of life often produce deathly conditions and obscure death and diverse forms of "letting die." Thus we follow the more Foucauldian line to focus on death as the *contingent underside* to the very means of pursuing and maximizing life, where the powers of death are exercised in the "exigencies of a life-administering power."[40] We focus, then, on such contingent operations: forms of vulnerability, death-in-life, and death effects that regularly accompany insistent life-making in liberal democratic regimes.

In this way, our work resonates with research on the racializing dimensions and politics of difference within liberal governance, neoliberal capitalism, and/or biomedicine, such as that offered by Anne Pollock in her analysis of race-based pharmaceuticals as *pharmakon*—both remedy and harbinger of danger within contemporary marketized healthscapes—and in the emerging literature on the uneven incorporation of marginalized subjects into neoliberal reproductive imperatives.[41] Exemplary of the latter is Grace Kyungwon Hong's work, which focuses on how select modes of minoritized life are invited into reproductive respectability in neoliberal times, precisely to disavow the ongoing and exacerbated production of premature death for others.[42] Such analysis complements this volume's focus on the ways subjects are called on to affirm life and participate in life-making protocols and activities that perpetuate inequities and frequently obfuscate their deathly effects and consequences. More generally, we draw inspiration from Orlando Patterson's important conceptualization of "social death"[43] and see this book connecting with such work as Lisa Marie Cacho's examination of the ways personhood and rights-based politics normalize social and literal death, specifically "the unchallenged devaluation of criminalized populations of color";[44] Lauren Berlant's formulation of "slow death" as the "destruction of life, bodies, imaginaries, and environments by and under contemporary regimes of capital";[45] Henry Giroux's discussion of the "biopolitics of disposability" and abjected racialized populations marked for death; Matthew Sparke's diagnostic of "biological subcitizenship" and the embodiment of ill health under austerity conditions; and Ruthie Gilmore's key theorization of racism as "the state-sanctioned or extralegal production and exploitation of group-differentiated vulnerability to premature death."[46]

Finally, this book considers alternative biocultures and "living on," by meditating on death and actions/activisms, policies, and practices that affirm other ways of living and dying—that are unfaithful to the governing logics that we analyze. Our ethical stance is focused on challenging modes of agency and how we are governed—through acknowledging, exploring, and valuing possibilities of "living on" within death-in-life. In contrast to studies of "affirmative biopolitics" that seek to reclaim the power of life from governmental structures—"flipping" the negative diagnosis of the violent and authoritarian potential of biopower—this book examines affirmation as a governing operation that is not inherently good or emancipatory: we do not reinterpret biopolitics affirmatively as a strategy of scholarly ethical intervention but rather scrutinize the complex relationships between "make live" and "let die" through the concrete case studies we present.[47] Additionally, an outflow of literature focused on "life" has implemented vitalist or "new materialist" approaches that problematize the boundaries of life and death, the human, nature, and so forth.[48] This project intersects with these approaches, in that we are interested in cells, the afterlife of dead bodies, or the vitality of cancer; however, we track the administration of materiality and politics of life—*not* vitality as an ethical base of life or affirmations of life outside the human. We similarly recognize the reverse ethical move of embracing the "death drive," such as that presented in Lee Edelman's work on the refusal of reproductive futurism, and/or rejecting the call to "make live" on the grounds that it produces deathly effects.[49] An example of the latter approach is Alastair Hunt and Stephanie Youngblood's edited volume, which proposes a humanities-led refusal of cultural affirmations of life. While the overall critical position of "against life"—to refuse to theorize collective politics under the sign of life—is important to consider, the effort potentially limits political engagement to a matter of "choice" (i.e., choosing to reject life) and assumes equal access to that subject position without addressing forms of death-in-life.[50]

In what follows, we do not privilege the life–death dyad but instead seek out the ways that life-making creates better chances for some and affords some people the capacity to pursue or reject more life. The core ethical imperative of this book, then, is to enhance our understanding of the ways people are positioned unequally within biomedicine and its logics, and of how extending more life (for some) obscures deadly inequities. Advancing ethics as a form of critique, in ways that seek to refashion the normative terms of existence, we ask, how might we endure in the contours of deadly life-making?

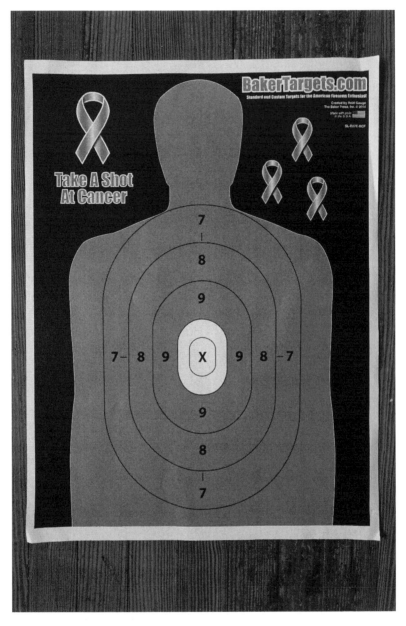

Figure 1. Breast cancer–customized firearm target poster. Photograph courtesy of the authors.

1

Hope

Cancer

Do you know what hope is? It's magic and it's free.
It's not in a prescription. It's not in an IV.
It punctuates our laughter. It sparkles in our tears.
It simmers under sorrows. It dissipates our fears.
Do you know what hope is? It's reaching past today.
It's dreaming of tomorrow. It's trying a new way.
It's questioning the answer. It's always seeking more.
It's rumors of a break. It's whispers of a cure.
A roller coaster ride. Of remedies, unsure.
Do you know what hope is? It's candy for the soul.
It's perfume for the spirit. To share it makes you whole.
Keep Hope Forever Until We Find A CURE.

—"Banners of Hope," *Sunshine after the Rain Blog*

It is within disease, with its terrifying phantoms of despair and hope that
my body becomes ripe as little else for encoding that which society holds to
be real.

—Michael Taussig, "Reification and the Consciousness of the Patient"

Hope carries utopian promise; it offers possibilities of a "not yet," a "to come," and an imagining of life otherwise. Hope has often been deployed as the means to effect radical social transformation and the reinvention of reality.[1] It is seen as a way of reaching beyond the stymied conditions of today by orienting toward the horizon of an alternative tomorrow. Hope is invoked as an incantation, under conditions of uncertainty, of the ability to effect change. This change can be imagined politically and economically, psychologically and corporeally. Indeed, hope is ubiquitous in contemporary culture, from then-U.S. President Barack Obama's political memoir *The Audacity of Hope* to international food drives—the "Convoy of Hope"[2]—

to biomedical understandings of illness and health. As in the preceding quotation from "Banners of Hope" (an online outreach for children with life-threatening diseases), hope is often the panacea for chronic or terminal illness.

Hope—to have hope, to show hope, to activate hope, to marshal hope—is viewed and pursued as ontologically "good," as unquestionably the right way to be/live. Yet, in the biocultural arena, the *affirmation of hope* (often taking the form of a demand *to* hope) operates in a regulatory sense to structure subjectivities, social realities, and corporeal states. Hope incites particular behaviors, it induces certain forms of community and belonging, and it encourages us to believe in the possible transcendence of bodily limits and/or temporal constraints. In contemporary U.S. biocultures of cancer specifically, hope operates as a form of intimate governance that conditions responses to bodily vulnerability and uncertainty and manages the present for the future.[3] In this chapter, we analyze how hope is articulated and employed in cancer activism and awareness campaigns, fund-raising, forms of treatment, and clinical spaces and practices to "make live." In looking to the ways the affirmation of hope is actively made and maintained in what we call *spectacles of hope, infrastructures of care,* and *bioethics of faith,* several limitations become evident. First, we see that only certain forms of hope are validated in cancer biocultures, and in late liberalism, these dominant affective conventions of hope are increasingly commodified, routinized, and militarized.[4] Second, while such dominant forms of hope orient individuals and the population at large toward life—indeed, dominant forms of hope relentlessly affirm life—the affirmation of hope also has death-effects: hope itself may not be deadly, but it can cover over death, distract us from seeing death-producing factors, and create or maintain deadly conditions for certain sectors of the population. We show that individuals who do not (or are not able to) embody dominant modes of hope—and thus fight cancer in a way that resounds in popular discourse—are framed as failed or negligent and invisibilized or abandoned within the cultural realm. Moreover, as we explore in the final part of the chapter, the insistence on hoping for the biomedical cure precludes a social justice approach that would actually apprehend the environmental, class-based, and racialized causes of cancer incidence. Hope discourse thus lets certain individuals/communities (continue to) die and can be seen to abandon individuals whose prognosis is "terminal." We ultimately ask, how can individuals find other ways to live with and die from cancer, not through forsaking hope, but through developing and practicing alternative hope tactics—"hoping for other things"—in relation to cancer?

The Affect of Hope in U.S. Biocultures

Affect refers to affections, sentiments, perceptions, and proclivities that circulate within and are produced through social and material/environmental relations.[5] Affect is actively constructed through representations, practices, and interpersonal relations: it is inextricable from social realities. Affect is socially and materially arranged and directed and is conditioned through sets of norms. These norms regarding certain affects (that regularize how to be sad, how to be happy, how to be angry, etc.) organize how we encounter one another and the world around us, and they call on us to generate and cultivate certain responses over others. As Clare Hemmings has noted, then, "affect might in fact be valuable [to criticism, to analysis] precisely to the extent that it is *not* autonomous."[6]

Multiple affects become solidified through practices and institutions. Importantly, certain affects are valued and socially endorsed; some affects become dominant and are normalized, while others remain subjugated and devalued. Furthermore, specific understandings or responses are seen as more acceptable than others within the contours of a particular affect. Norms of a given affect constrain (or mark the limits of) knowledge and experience of that affect. These complexities call for a nuanced approach to the analysis of affect, one that takes into account the manifold social implications of affective norms and their material effects. Such an investigation is necessary because of the differential ways that norms of a given affect are productive: forming and conditioning bodies, subjectivities, and broader group identities and social relations. The stakes of conceptualizing affect as social (rather than ontological) are that politics remains embedded in embodied subjects and the practices of everyday life.

Within contemporary biocultures, hope is clearly a dominant affect. Many critical studies of biomedicine and technoscience fields have analyzed the nuanced workings of hope—its operations at individual and broader social levels: Mary-Jo Delvecchio-Good et al. have analyzed what they termed the "political economy of hope" in oncology culture; Sarah Franklin has examined new reproductive technologies as "technologies of hope"; Tiago Moreira and Paolo Palladino have investigated the tensions and mutual relations between what they call the "regimes of hope and truth"; and Carlos

Novas has built on the idea of a political economy of hope by applying it to the analysis of links between corporations, individuals, and the production of biovalue. Nik Brown's sustained attention to hope has drawn together multiple scholars working in this area of inquiry and, further, extended understandings of how hope is mediated in biomedicine, specifically in terms of biomedical expectations.[7]

This is not to say that other affects—such as despair, shame, fear, and anger—are unimportant: multiple affects *do* permeate biomedical encounters and broader collective and individual responses to illness within biocultural spheres. However, other affects are not actively fostered in biomedical engagements or in broader social articulations of disease and illness in the ways that hope is. Importantly, hope—in its dominance—operates as a form of *intimate governance*: it conditions particular ways of living, at the level both of the population and of the individual, and is thus both biopolitical and disciplinary. Hope works biopolitically in that it is rhetorically invoked and utilized across a broad spectrum of biomedical practices, formal biomedical institutions, and social infrastructures to orient the population toward more life. Hope operates as a form of discipline in the sense that individuals are encouraged to hope as the way to affirm their own life: hope is integral to the regulation of the self and individual bodies.

The "productivity" of hope—its uptake and its biopolitical and disciplinary effects—should *not,* however, be equated with widespread support for diverse forms of hope. Following on from our earlier point, like other affects, hope is conventionalized in particular ways that circumscribe what meanings or articulations of hope can exist and how hope is employed and experienced within biomedicine and contemporary biocultures. These conventions reveal the power relations at work within affective states and practices of hope: hope disciplines individuals to affirm (a circumscribed) life—to experience their biomedical subjectivity through conventions of hope and to hope *as* the way to live (more). One of the primary ways that hope has been conventionalized is through biomedicine itself—through biomedical encounters that condition individual feelings and responses to medical treatments and expertise. Hope affirms the "truths" that undergird biomedicine.[8] These might be understood as the following: techno-utopian transcendentalism, or the possibility of transcendence of corporeal limits and ends; progress to an undefined future; a salvationary ethics that directs toward optimism; and optimization and enhancement of the human.[9] By affirming these truths central to biomedicine, hope fosters life in particular ways and encourages certain ways of thinking about life (in the face of illness). The biomedical deployment of hope orients life toward these truths and, in doing so, conditions conduct and produces biomedical subjects in line with biopolitical rationalities of life-making. Importantly, however, because affect—as it operates in biocultures—is connected to broader social events, such as the economy and national policy, biocultural conventions of hope shift over time. In other words, hope becomes conventionalized in ways that delimit how hope is embodied and practiced, *but* these conventions (the ways hope is imagined) also shift over time in relation to economic, political, social, and scientific developments.

To explore these claims further, we turn to an analysis of hope in relation to cancer. Historically, hope has played a key role in the public address of cancer in the United States. The shame, dread, fears of contagion, and embarrassment that attended individual discoveries of cancer perpetuated its social concealment and a general repugnance to the disease.[10] According to Susan Sontag, these sentiments toward cancer originated in large part because "cancer is notorious for attacking parts of the body (colon, bladder, rectum, breast, cervix, prostate, testicles) that are embarrassing to acknowledge."[11] To battle cancer's stigma, hope was purposely cultivated and conscripted as a counteraffect to raise public awareness of cancer and rally public resources for cancer prevention and treatment. This was—and continues to be—filtered through militarized rhetoric and practice, evidenced most clearly by the historic mobilization of hope as a weapon in the "war on cancer."[12] Among the linkages between cancer and militarism (for example, chemotherapy drugs and biochemical warfare[13]), hope weaponry has operated in both a discursive sense and in practice through the political economy of treatment of cancer and broader public cancer campaigns and services. These militant operations of hope are more observable in some cancer activisms than others, for example, breast cancer compared to bladder cancer, but all cancers are, to some degree, managed and represented through vigilant biocultural deployments of hope—its relays and forays through biomedicine and into the public realm. In the following section, we briefly survey the rise of hope as the militant affirmation of life within cancer activism, specifically the weaponizing of hope in breast cancer culture, which dramatically emblematizes the intensified deathly potential of the contemporary pursuit of life against cancer. We consider some of the changing conventions of hope within the war on cancer to open up a broader discussion of the ways this affect governs within biocultures of cancer—both mobilizing and limiting life through various terrains of cancer activism and treatment.

Hope Weaponry in the War on Cancer

Cancer has long been considered the target of war—that which war must be waged against—with hope serving as a primary weapon to fight cancer. Hope was first deployed in biocitizenship projects relating to cancer in the late nineteenth and early twentieth centuries.[14] During this time, a generalized silence accompanied the disease, and there was an overriding popular belief that a cancer diagnosis inevitably resulted in death. Despite high incidence and mortality rates, cancer received little public attention. To battle these issues and work toward the goal of the promotion of life, public education efforts and a series of social-control programs endeavored to "fight cancer with publicity" and combat the fear and silence surrounding it with hope. The American Society for the Control of Cancer (the ASCC, which became the American Cancer Society [ACS]) formally adopted the Sword of Hope symbol in 1928. The sword was used to promote the idea that vigilant detection, knowledge, and education would enable individuals to hope that they would not succumb to cancer but could instead battle it and thus make themselves live.[15] Hope, in this era, was beginning to be militarized; it was considered the battle cry to wage war on cancer, and the sword rallied hope to encourage individuals to take responsibility for their own health and that of their families, and to discipline themselves with the aim of achieving national protection against cancer.[16]

Integral to the rising public visibility of cancer was the formation of the Women's Field Army (WFA). Established in 1936 and initiated by the ASCC, the WFA adopted the Sword of Hope as its emblem and aimed to collectively organize "trench warfare with a vengeance against a ruthless killer."[17] Organized vertically with an officer's corps and foot volunteers, enlisted women in this legion of volunteers wore khaki uniforms with insignias of rank and achievement. By 1943, the WFA numbered between 350,000 and 700,000 and was supported by militarized forms of hope within popular culture, such as posters that exhorted citizens to vanquish cancer by learning about it, looking for symptoms, and pursuing early diagnosis and treatment as part of a collective front against cancer.[18] While various medico-technical advancements were unfolding during this time period, the strength of national health relied on individual and familial efforts to promote cancer awareness and retaliation against the disease. Cancer was seen as a disease that could be controlled by knowing its symptoms and anticipating its signs, and thus both hope and cancer's curability relied on early detection once the disease had appeared. The aim, here, was to regularize the lives of the masses (in line with normative standards) and mitigate the risks faced by the population at large. This possibility could only be mobilized through the militancy of citizens over their own bodies and those of their families; to do otherwise meant that one failed as a citizen. The Sword of Hope was a call to arms in this enterprise, where the conquest of cancer was framed as a civic duty, a matter of honor, and a heroic endeavor that required the vigilance of the entire population.

In contemporary biocultures of cancer, hope operates differently. First, hope remains central to governing, but it now involves a heightened individual triumphalism bolstered by popular and biomedical efforts to optimize life, to make (individuals) live (more). Hope is no longer positioned as a social and collective expression of national belonging and welfare but is instead framed as something potentially embodied in one's own biological material and facilitated by biotech advancements and corporations. Massive investment in the life sciences and biotechnologies from the 1970s onward has effectively led to a political economy of life that speculates on life and its possibilities—in contradistinction to the earlier period's regularizing of life and collectivizing of risk. Biomedicine has extended its terrain from illness to the more all-encompassing and pervasive regime of "health"; it has increasingly customized rather than normalized the body and, through the genetic and molecular framing of life, promoted preemption and militant self-care in place of an overarching sense of national belonging and protection.[19] Attendant to these biomedical shifts, hope is now marshalled as a personal—rather than primarily collective—refusal of death.

Second, fighting *through hope* in the war against cancer—as seen in the endless pursuit of the biomedical cure and cancer awareness campaigns— is now heavily corporatized and commodified. Breast cancer activism, in particular, has witnessed the corporatization and commercialization of hope weaponry. Breast cancer currently receives more coverage than any other type of cancer, and hope permeates almost all rhetoric and practices that surround the disease.[20] Breast cancer is the disease that inspires— *demands*—the most hope, and such hypervisible hope has been largely achieved through the commercialization of breast cancer activism. In distinction from earlier cancer activism and control programs that emphasized civic responsibility, cancer awareness drives and fund-raising are now heavily directed through corporate sponsorship and take place in/through the market and what Barbara Ehrenreich and other critics have called the *cancer–industrial complex.*[21] This is readily apparent in the contemporary linkages between breast cancer activism and drug manufacturers, such as AstraZeneca. This company's predecessor, Imperial Chemical Industries, initiated National Breast Cancer Awareness Month (in 1985, in partnership with the ACS), the largest vehicle for cancer-related activism in the world. Breast cancer reveals the extent to which education, activism, and marketing have blurred under the banner of hope. For example, the pervasive color known as "breast cancer pink" allows for the expression of awareness and support for breast cancer activism through pink branding ("pinkwashing") and consumerism. Hope is now key to making breast and other cancers palatable through the conventions of the commodity.[22]

The Walther P-22 Hope edition handgun captures these significant shifts of hope in biomedicine and beyond as they relate to cancer. Discount Gun Sales, a U.S. gun-manufacturing company, produced a limited number of special-edition pistols sporting a pink DuraCoat finish. They were introduced during Breast Cancer Awareness Month in 2011 with the original intention of donating a portion of the sales proceeds to the Susan G. Komen Foundation for breast cancer research.[23] The gun was so successful that, in 2012, the company initiated a second production line. A Hope edition breast cancer pink handgun is merely one product in a wide array of commodities within cancer popular culture and activism wherein hope functions as an affective currency—hope is bought and sold. By buying the breast cancer handgun (or any other kind of hope paraphernalia), one participates in a market of/for hope: one buys into a system of optimism and consumer identification—an economy sponsored by corporate bodies—to show support for the cause. However, the hope gun's death-making potential is absurdly drafted in the service of the cure for breast cancer. The gun rallies the war on cancer as a literal technology of killing that couples militant preemption with the normative femininity of pink-ribbon campaigns. While the anti–breast cancer handgun is an extreme example, it is not far afield from one of the dominant figures in contemporary U.S. breast cancer culture: the "pink warrior," a highly individualized and triumphalist symbol of resistance to breast cancer. This militant pink hero rallies public hope and optimism to combat the threat of cancer in or through commodified images and ideas of a certain form of feminism—

universalized sisterhood, self-empowerment, girl power, and so forth.[24] The "princess gear" associated with this emblematic figure shows how the militarization of breast cancer operates through masculinized conventions and norms that paradoxically work to recuperate "womanness" and promotes the ideal breast cancer patient as simultaneously infantilized and militarized. The pink warrior's call for militant hope and retaliation against breast cancer "combines with the saccharine commercial aspects of corporate breast cancer culture—the pink teddy bears, pink jelly beans, and so forth—to produce a spectacle of fanatical sugar-coated warfare."[25]

Third, this militant hope in breast cancer culture—exemplified by the Hope handgun—dovetails with a more general hypervigilant biomedicalized approach to the individual body and everyday life in contemporary times.[26] Advancements in biotechnology—the "march of progress" to current forms of genetic testing—have initiated new understandings of the body and practices of self-care (forms of individual discipline) that emphasize both individual genetic risk and health as a continuum. Departing significantly from the earlier era's curative model of disease, the paradigm has now shifted from cancer's curability after evidence of disease to a new form of life—the search for "the cure"—that involves endless detection and prediagnostic subjection to potential disease. Life, then, exists within a "pre-vivor" to "survivor" loop, and health has become an endless and hypervigilant individual enterprise. Breast cancer surveillance, in particular, through the historical mounting of biotechnologies, from the pap smear in the 1940s to the mammogram in the 1960s and genetic testing in the 1980s, has become a speculative and endless quest for the cure, to the extent that militant medical disciplining of the body through disease surveillance now traverses all stages of life. For example, there have been proposals to remove the breast buds of girl children who test positive for the BRCA1/ BRCA2 breast cancer genes.[27] The cure for breast cancer is, therefore, biomedically illusive, in that it defers any possibility for the "end" of cancer by enfolding persons without symptoms, along with unwanted and unknown futures, into the present in the name of cancer preemption. The idea of the cure rallies individuals around the pursuit of more life by obliging them to subject themselves to efforts of detection and optimization, thus extending the pursuit of the cure throughout everyday life. The hope gun is the ultimate fetish of this militant affirmation of life through constant preemptive action: "I will refuse death." As a breast cancer pink–themed object, the gun's operation now commemorates the higher purpose of breast cancer's cause, obfuscating the terror and death associated with both the actual disease and the gun itself. In doing this, the hope gun shows the complete depoliticization of "life" under the banner of optimizing (one's own) life; even the specter of death—via the technology of the gun—can be peddled as hope for the cure, as hope for more life.

While we do not mean to suggest that the hope gun serves as the ultimate public image for cancer or the paradigmatic icon of hope in contemporary U.S. biocultures of cancer, its existence captures the extent to which the governing of life has changed: the war on cancer and search for the cure now extend into previously untapped aspects of everyday life, and hope is militarized to such a degree that affirming life equates to pursuing and morally justifying individual security at any cost. From the hope sword of an earlier era of cancer control and prevention to a handgun that directs its preemptive violence toward "kicking cancer's ass," the call to hope organizes how individuals come to incorporate biomedical truths and rationalities—and biopolitical logics—in their daily lives. By incorporating these truths, individuals are not simply inert or consenting targets of biomedical power/knowledge and governance but "are always also the elements of its articulation."[28] We are now witnessing the emergence of new forms of citizenship where individuals increasingly think of themselves in relation to their biological, genetic, or corporeal status and discipline themselves accordingly.[29] If life is now understood as that which can be endlessly enhanced, optimized, customized, commodified, and biologized, then hope is articulated—and comes to be embodied—as the refusal to be limited to biological capacity and the way to speculate on one's own life, and life in general. Hope is the relentless optimism and demand for more (individual) life, the hypervigilance required of disease detection, and the militant affirmation of the endless productivity and potential of biotechnology and biomedical advancements. In the next section, we turn to the ways that conventions of hope are practiced and enacted across a diverse biocultural terrain—what we map out as spectacle, care, and faith—to explore how individuals come to incorporate biomedical truths and logics in their daily lives. By examining how hope operates within public representations of cancer, clinical settings, and encounters—across various scales of private to public, individual body to collectives, home to the clinic—we can see how the affect of hope contours life in particular ways and how such operations either obfuscate death or have deathly effects.

Spectacle, Care, and Faith: Terrains of Hope in Cancer Biocultures

Spectacles of Hope

The affirmation to hope has flourished through the proliferation of spectacles of hope within U.S. cancer biocultures of the twenty-first century. Via spectacle, biomedical rationales are endorsed and hope is continually mobilized and reenergized. This takes place through paraphernalia, in merchandizing, and in the paroxysm of mass cancer-centered events. Ultimately, such spectacles of hope structure what we should *hope for* in relation to cancer and how that hope should look.

Hope is most commonly turned into a spectacle via commodity items—such as the hope gun—that are adorned with imagery, branding, and slogans that represent the dominant way this affect has been conditioned in the biocultural arena. These items might be thought of as "hope paraphernalia" that enter hope into the market as a sentiment, orientation, and aesthetic that can be peddled and consumed. The spectacle embodied by these items calls on individuals to participate in the circulation of endless and affirmative hope through consumption and visual display: buying and displaying these tokens of hope come to represent an individual's commitment to either supporting the war more generally—in line with dominant understandings of life, health, and illness—or fighting that war on the personal front through what is known as survivorship. One can purchase hope-themed cancer awareness–raising products, such as mugs decaled with the slogan "Got Hope? I Do"; dog outfits that sport the caption "Love, Hope, and Peace"; a panoply of T-shirts emblazoned with motivational maxims such as "Wish, Hope, Love, and a Cure"; and bracelets labeled with "Hope" and "Strength." You can quite literally carry hope by buying a LeSportsac Hope Garden or Miche Premium Shell Hope handbag or wear hope in the form of a piece of eternity-symbol jewelry called the Hope Band.[30] Organic life can be instrumentalized in the service of hope and the breast cancer cause through the purchase of Hope SeedBallz, which enable you to "plant an all-pink garden."[31] Moreover, the spectacle of hope has extended into the global market such that in Sweden, for instance, one can figuratively buy and gift hope to someone with cancer through purchasing the Give Hope Box—an empty box full of hope, the proceeds from which are donated to childhood cancer.[32]

The spectacle of hope also predominates in the slogans for cancer awareness and fund-raising, as evidenced by the basketball fund-raiser named
Hoops 4 Hope,[33] the art-based cancer initiative Boards of Hope (which
"invites artists to transform recycled boards of all types into canvases for
stunning works of art, based on the theme, *Healing & Hope*"[34]), and the
Ulman Cancer Fund for Young Adults, whose beer- and wine-tasting fund-
raising events are advertised under the slogan "Screw Cancer, Brew Hope."
Cancer-focused organizations equally draw from and reproduce the spec-
tacle of hope through advertising and various initiatives. For instance, the
ACS's Relay for Life website greets the viewer with information on what the
ACS calls Heroes of Hope, and Livestrong has Hope Rides and supports
Fertile Hope for cancer patients. Not only evident in these arenas, the spectacle of hope (as the answer or appropriate response to cancer) has been
co-opted by the broader market to become a vehicle for sales. The Breast
Cancer Action group Think Before You Pink warns that, while seemingly
altruistic, the "companies know that aligning themselves with 'breast cancer
awareness' will improve the public's perception of them and increase their
profits."[35] Accordingly, an advertising campaign such as Hyundai's Hope on
Wheels—where you can buy a car and the manufacturer will supply what
it calls a "hope grant" to a child with cancer—needs to be understood as a
spectacle within the cancer–corporate–market nexus.[36]

Mass events and rallies for cancer represent perhaps the most powerful form of hope as spectacle. Of these, the Susan G. Komen Race for the
Cure and the Avon Walk for Breast Cancer are conceivably the most well
known and spectacular. According to Komen advertising, their race is "the
world's largest and most successful education and fundraising event for
breast cancer *ever created*,"[37] and more than 130 Komen events per year
are organized globally. Avon holds walks in nine U.S. cities throughout
the year and calls participants into the cause with the slogan "2 days and
39 miles of unstoppable hope." Like other forms of cancer-hope spectacle,
however, these events cannot be divorced from the commodification of cancer. They are corporate-sponsored, and as Ehrenreich has noted, "the Avon
Breast Cancer Crusade . . . spends more than a third of the money raised
on overhead and advertising, and Komen may similarly fritter away up to
25 percent of its gross."[38] Such events cannot be extricated from the ways
these organizations may be implicated in producing deaths. For instance,
Avon sponsors the Look Good . . . Feel Better program (that runs beauty
workshops for women undergoing breast cancer treatment), yet more than

250 of the makeup and other products used in the program have been listed on a health risk database in the highest concern category "due to the presence of hormone disruptors, neurotoxins, and possible carcinogens."[39] And both organizations promote mammography as a first-line defense in disease detection, which many have criticized as leading to overdiagnosis and unnecessary treatment, including surgery, radiation, and exposure to potentially toxic and deadly drugs.[40]

Yet both of these mass events invite individuals to create an enduring spectacle of hope through various techniques: solidarity in walking/running for the cause; the adornment of pink-themed clothing, pom-poms, and other paraphernalia; and the use of anthems and theme songs. Importantly, however, it must be noted that such events enlist women who have already come to think of themselves as "citizens of breast cancer," who have been disciplined to think of the disease as a property of their individuality, and who relate to the disease through a highly individualized framing of hope. This individualization might best be seen in one of Komen's key slogans: "I am the cure." Rallies, then, massify the individual militancy to hope through collective spectacle. In turn, the events become powerful conduits for and of hope, which is framed as the affect that enables one to "be energized, be inspired."[41] Thus these events operate as *disciplinary technologies,* in that they actively foster the dominant operations of hope as relentless optimism and future thinking. This optimism, as Ehrenreich has powerfully argued, "celebrat[es] survivorhood by downplaying mortality."[42] Indeed, it *eclipses* the struggle with uncertainty that is situated at the center of being diagnosed with breast cancer and obscures both death and the fact that cancer haunts society. As Dorothy Broom laments in her own account of breast cancer, "no widows weeds, no black armbands, no ritual keening, shaved heads or body paint distinguish the bereaved [in mass spectacles]."[43] Sarah Polzin Schultz, a stage IV breast cancer patient, similarly remarks in her online commentary on the alienating effects of hope-as-survivorship, "The definition of 'survivor' is: a person who remains alive in an event where others have died. How does that apply to the incurable?"[44] The spectacle of hope might, in this sense, operate as cruel optimism.[45]

Infrastructures of Care

It is difficult to imagine any form of cancer care not predicated on hope. The sustained marriage between *care* and *hope* constitutes the very essence of countless cancer treatment spaces and practices that regard fostering hope to be integral to providing care. The pursuit of hope as an operation of care is well established and continues to set the stage for biomedical encounters: people interface with biomedicine in/through care services that aver hope. In the contemporary era, hope is intensively fostered, and the subject governed, through architectures of care that instrumentalize interior design and customize medical services in the cause of hope—in other words, the increased efficiency and corporatization of care, combined with hope *thematics*. Numerous hospitals, medical centers, and cancer treatment hubs employ hope in their titles, such as City of Hope in Los Angeles, one of forty National Cancer Institute–designated comprehensive cancer treatment centers. Hope medical care titles also have a global presence, demonstrated by the numerous North American examples beyond the borders of the United States, such as the Breast Cancer Center of Hope in Manitoba, Canada, and the Oasis of Hope Cancer Hospital in Tijuana, Mexico. Many of these treatment centers strive to integrate cancer care services—blood tests, scans, chemotherapy sessions, and other support provisions—under one roof. Hope is generated through the efficiencies of a coordinated and comprehensive infrastructure of care. The integration of different offices and services reduces patient travel and allows for enhanced customization of care. Treatment centers organize doctors and medical service professionals into "care teams" that collaborate and tailor procedures according to each patient's needs. The patient is thus treated as an individual fulcrum of hope that can be leveraged by a care team, well-organized services, and effective architecture.

Beyond teamwork tailored to each patient and the fostering of hope through architectural efficiencies, cancer care centers also seek to cultivate hope through spatial arrangements and decor. Treatment centers increasingly attempt to embody hope—hope as inspirational, calm, compassionate, and optimistic care—in their very architectural designs and interiors. For example, the Mission Hope Cancer Center in Santa Maria, California, which opened in late April 2012, offers "comprehensive compassionate cancer care" within one three-story, 44,000-square-foot building, featuring a Mediterranean-style architectural exterior with natural landscaping and vistas of the surrounding valley.[46] The interior design includes external windows that pool warm, natural light; spacious seating rooms in earth tones; large ceiling portals that brighten enclosed rooms with back-lit images of blue sky; and enlarged nature photographs that serve as kiosk screens, room dividers, and window shades and that express light as natural shading. Surf photography dons many of the walls, to exude color and motivational flourishes; expansive windows overlooking the Santa Maria Valley serve as backdrop to the administration of chemotherapy on the third floor; and patients undergoing various scans and procedures can gaze on vividly back-lit, majestic landscape images that have been incorporated into the ceilings. Such hope theming, particularly the enlarged nature transparencies, creates a calming and contemplative "aquarium-bowl" effect; one potentially feels better about one's disease or illness on viewing inspirational nature at every interface within the medical establishment. Mission Hope Cancer Center's "nature-sanctuary" interior design conditions patients to admire nature, feel comfortable, be positive, and pursue treatment of oneself as part of the larger flourishing of life.

A second example, the University of Arkansas for Medical Sciences Winthrop P. Rockefeller Cancer Institute in Little Rock, debuted, in 2010, a twelve-story, 300,000-square-foot expansion for cancer research, treatment, and outreach. The design of the entire building was carefully considered as a means to inspire the hope of patients and their families.[47] The interior holds numerous hope-themed environmental attributes: wall-displayed affirmations like "While there's life, there's hope," live piano playing, and an atrium housing a garden and the *Seed of Hope* sculpture—the hallmark of the entire building.[48] Carved from white-pearl Turkish marble and standing two feet high, this sculpture of a large seed serves as a dedicated monumental receptacle for Seed of Hope tokens.[49] Such tokens, which feature the logo of the institute on one side and an impression of the interior of a seed on the other, are presented to patients on the final day of their active cancer treatment. Each patient is given two seed coins: one token is placed in the sculpture to commemorate survivorship, and the other is taken home by the patient to keep or to gift to another person as a symbol of hope.[50] In this scenario, the affirmation of/to hope is symbolically minted in monetary-coin form and pressed into the service of an expansive, contemplative, timeless, and copyrighted landscape of cancer care, extending from the sculpture itself to the larger building surrounding the atrium and sculpture and to the pockets and homes of cancer patients and their relations. Such an affective economy encourages the cultural acceptance of cancer through the visually encouraging accumulation of hope; it also primes individuals to accept, internalize, and advertise corporatized forms of care.

The contemporary corporatization of cancer care—and the contradictions that attend it—can be further explored through examination of the ACS-administered Hope Lodge network. Various Hope Lodges have been built in urban centers across the United States. Each offers cancer patients and their caregivers invaluable free, temporary lodging when specialized cancer treatments are unavailable near their homes. Hope Lodges also offer many practical services and infrastructures essential to everyday life to reduce the financial and emotional burdens of cancer treatment: guest rooms and private baths, common kitchens, computer workstations, a library with educational material on hand, local transportation to and from treatment, and additional communal opportunities, including yoga, Tai Chi, and shared meals.[51] Such care employs the architecture and interior environment to nurture hope, homelike comfort, private retreat, and community connection. With more than thirty locations bearing the official trademarked name, Hope Lodges serve and simulate community welfare—especially critical in the context of the U.S. market-driven health care "system," which provides few guarantees and limited custody of those facing illness and disease. The provision of this hope network presents corporations an opportunity to articulate hope through corporate benevolence, such as AstraZeneca's donation of $7 million for the founding of the Hope Lodge in Boston in 2006, now accordingly named the "AstraZeneca Hope Lodge Center."[52] Similar to what critics have called "greenwashing," corporate sponsorship can strategically function as *carewashing*—drawing attention to corporate social responsibility in one corner, while irresponsible and harmful practices continue elsewhere.[53] The parent company of AstraZeneca, for instance, manufactures carcinogenic insecticides and pesticides. AstraZeneca itself produces the breast cancer treatment drugs tamoxifen and Amiradex, and tamoxifen has been identified as a known carcinogen (causing ovarian cancer) by the U.S. National Institutes of Health. Effectively, then, such companies can harm—indeed, potentially kill—the bodies of those they are claiming to help. And rather than contributing to the marginalized research on the environmental causes of cancer, which could potentially implicate corporations like AstraZeneca and their predecessor companies, hopeful architectures and networks of care could be seen to Band-Aid over the cancer–industrial complex,[54] obfuscating potential hazards and harms that commence or continue under the banner of corporate benevolence *and* the intensified reliance upon corporate charity as the arena and conduit for medical care.

Bioethics of Faith

Beyond being pursued and fostered in practices of spectacle and care, hope also operates in biocultures of cancer as a form of faith. U.S. oncology, most specifically, is permeated by a discourse of *hope as faith* in biomedicine, in the self, and in the affirmation of life.[55] Such hope refuses the limits of life and calls on subjects to become active participants that instrumentalize the future, discipline themselves to be hopeful, and maintain faith in biomedical progress. While Western science and medicine historically can be seen to supersede religious truth and salvation with a *telos* of progress, current techno-utopian orientations toward biotechnologies, attendant to shifts within biomedicine from simply control (of disease and of populations) to customization and participation, have made hope a *bioethics of faith*—an ethical orientation predicated on the pursuit of salvation—that prompts subjects to internalize the pursuit of hope and marshal faith in the endless affirmation of life.

This bioethics of faith is most clearly seen in the tension that often exists between disclosure—a historically won patients' "right to know"—and the practical need to maintain patient cooperation with treatment regimes and what has been called the "principle of respect for hope."[56] Although hope has been criticized as providing justification for paternalism, the withholding of information, and other harms within the biomedical realm, the *full* disclosure of diagnosis can also be interpreted as medically inappropriate if it jeopardizes hope. Prognostic ambiguity and uncertainty, then, are the grounds on which disclosing and withholding of information are negotiated in the name of securing and managing hope. Within oncology, a dedicated interest in fostering hope can subvert the medical imperative of full disclosure (at the core of medical ethics), particularly when prognoses are bleak, with "facts as the killing fields."[57] When truth is not a productive means to manage patients, oncology enlists hope as an active therapeutic tool that orients patients to the future, affirms life, and rallies faith in the pursuit of always-more medical possibilities. Some even consider the oncologist's vocation to be instilling hope, balancing the obligation to be honest with "an equally important duty to cultivate hope."[58] Hope is understood to be transformative, potent, even capable of influencing the biological course of cancer; patients, therefore, have a right to it. The right to hope is intimately tied to U.S.-based notions of effective personhood and faith in the ability of individuals to shape life and corporeal functions through the power of will.[59]

This "allegiance to the efficacy of personal volition and the capacity of the self to mobilize a 'desire for life,' a 'will to live' and a 'fighting spirit'" is evident in the development and use of hope scales since the 1970s.[60] These instruments of psychometric measurement use affect for intense scrutiny, surveillance, and objectification. Specifically, they provide a means of assessing how much hope an individual has through establishing and deploying norms of acceptable levels of hope. The hope scales involve the administration of a carefully crafted series of questions that are then scored. Several scales are currently in existence, each exhibiting different nuances and backed by an expansive research network dedicated to the quantitative study of the hopeful properties of cancer patients.[61] As a whole, these hope diagnostics bifurcate psyche and soma, compelling subjects to monitor and regulate the psyche in order to heal the body. They substantiate hope as central to extended survival, harmonize patients with the aspirations of treatment programs, and, by splitting the psyche and soma, foster belief in the responsibility of the individual to gather "the necessary affective resources in overcoming personalized pathology."[62] Hope, however, is essentially pathologized through such hope scales, and subjects are held accountable for hope's absence—and disciplined to actively cultivate it.

Another way that individuals are called on to hope as a form of faith is through participating in virtual games that are designed to impart knowledge to patient-players about disease and treatments, rehearse medical protocols, and cultivate faith in self-efficacy. The nonprofit organization HopeLab, which engages in consumer-centered product development "to enhance the physical health and psychological well-being of young people with chronic diseases," brought together video game designers, health psychologists, and cancer researchers to design a game for young people with cancer.[63] The intention was to create and market a game that equipped patient-players with motivational and transformative affective experiences in order to practice vigilant self-care through virtually battling their disease. The result was a Microsoft Windows–based, third-person shooter game—*Re-mission*—released in 2006 with twenty-plus levels of gameplay. *Re-mission* immerses players within the complex, microscopic world of cancer-ridden bodies in an epic battle against cancer, wherein one's weapons are upgraded and more life is achieved by adhering to protocols of prescribed medications, timely symptom reporting, and side-effect management.[64] In the game, patient-players pilot a sassy nanobot named Roxxi through the cellular level of teenaged cancer patients to investigate symptoms, destroy cancer cells, stop metastases, and activate patients into "chemo compliance."[65] Players live out the contingencies of treatment in the game's virtual organic proving grounds. For example, if a patient skips chemotherapy doses, then Roxxi's chemo-concentrating blaster misfires every third shot and the cancer cells survive and become drug resistant. Considered a flagship for the health-gaming movement, with reportedly more than 185,000 copies distributed free of charge across eighty-one countries, the game has undergone controlled trials to measure its impact on patient behavior, and, based on these results, is said to have stimulated an increase in positive cancer-related attitudes by "transforming mundane medication into bullets to kill the enemy cells, and by changing the humdrum routine of swallowing pills into a heroic act."[66] Essentially, subjects internalize the dominant conventions of hope through the game's rehearsal of highly militaristic and individualistic self-care. By playing the game, subjects rally faith in biomedicine and, through techno-utopian transcendence, affirm life, the power of the self, and martial values. *Re-mission* activates a powerful exercise of militarized faith in self-efficacy and, in doing so, secures both the individualized disciplining of hope and the biopolitical optimization (of a certain form) of living.

Spiritual guidance around cancer treatment is a third area where hope as faith proliferates, as a joint venture of medical and religious communities. The integration of various spiritual diagnostics and services in the formal clinical process of treatment—what is often referred to as a *holistic* approach—increasingly dominates the field of cancer care. Regardless of the faith-based religious content at work in different cases, the biomedical protocol of oncology to foster hope and affirm life interestingly dovetails with religious practice. For example, research has been under way on the hypothesis that individuals with spiritual struggle have greater mortality, and the reverse, that spirituality heals and faith is "medicine's neglected spirit."[67] While biomedicine could be said to use religion to generate hope, the reverse could also be asserted. Religious communities have been engaged in biomedicine throughout the history of health care in the United States. Religiously affiliated hospitals and treatment centers, for instance, have a long-standing formal presence, especially Christian-oriented care and charity. What is new, however, are the explicit promotional claims and niche businesses of customized spiritual medical care that are taking place within the competitive health care market. The Cancer Treatment Centers of America (CTCA) emblematizes this significant trend, advertising their provision of "mind–body medicine," spiritual guidance, and a "mother standard of care," along with cutting-edge biotechnologies and treatment programs.[68] CTCA's "care that never quits" slogan asserts interminable care as the means to enduring hope, and its highly visible marketing strategy emphasizes the integration of medical faith and spiritual custodianship—that spiritual faith is vital to battling cancer.[69]

A related though less readily apparent facet of the CTCA is its Our Journey of Hope spiritual-support program, which advocates the communion of faith in care and healing with faith in God.[70] This salvationary enterprise, which portends to establish relations between medical and spiritual communities ("when religion and medicine embrace"), not only indicates a competitive strategy within the neoliberal marketplace of health care—the niche of serving spiritual hope and guidance—but also structures individual relations with biomedicine in such a way that patients have an opportunity to be born again through biomedical encounters, to heal themselves through relations with God and renewed Christian faith and optimism.[71] This extends individual self-care beyond the biological foundations of the human to *vigilance through God*. Religion compounds the biomedical affirmation of life to proliferate hope: if biomedical faith is hope in biomedicine to affirm biological life, then its combination with faith in God expands hope's *telos* beyond life and death. This expansion of affirmation beyond life and death, however, means that individuals now bear intensified moral and social responsibility to get healthy through God, matched with biomedical advancements. An article posted in the resources section of the CTCA's Our Journey of Hope website, "Don't Waste Your Cancer," implores readers to see their illnesses as a productive enterprise of faith: "you will waste your cancer if you do not believe it is designed for you by God.... You will waste your cancer if you believe it is a curse and not a gift.... You will waste your cancer if you seek comfort from your odds rather than from God.... You will waste your cancer if you grieve as those who have no hope."[72] To do otherwise—"to waste your cancer"—is not mere failure to enhance and optimize one's life; it is the fault of individuals—and individuals are deserving of death—for not attending to spiritual care, for not having faith in God, for not allowing cancer to teach them how to be hopeful. The title of another

CTCA-posted article alludes to this final judgment and the anathema that is death under the evangelical biomedical banner of endless hope: "Atheist Doctors More Likely to Hasten Death."[73]

Hoping for Other Things: Alternative Hope Tactics

As evidenced through the various practices of spectacle, care, and faith, the affect of hope (and affirmation to hope) has a pervasive governing function in U.S. biocultures of cancer. It is deployed in ways that support the biopolitical focus on affirming and enhancing the life of the population and increasingly structures the way that individuals are governed. This claim is clearly substantiated through the example of cancer culture, wherein hope directs an optimistic orientation to the future and to life, often predicated on militant organization and consumption. Hope is promoted and pursued and comes to function as a regulatory affect, disciplining social engagements with and individual responses to cancer: it affirms life, and this affirming relentlessly circumscribes the kind of life that can be lived and the forms of hope that are socially celebrated and endorsed.

This affirmation of life through hope is an intervening into life, a promoting of life. However, not all forms of life are fostered equally. Race, class, and sexuality—as they intersect with gender—heavily condition disease incidence and survival rates for cancer: economically disadvantaged, non-heterosexual, and racial and ethnic minorities are diagnosed later, receive disparities in care, and experience higher mortality rates in relation to cancer.[74] Moreover, the pursuit of well-being and optimal health has largely become a privatized concern dependent on social status, including educational background, financial means, and racially and ethnically stratified access to care and resources. According to the National Cancer Institute's race/ethnic categorizations, African Americans/blacks, Asian Americans, Hispanics, American Indians, Alaska Natives, and underserved whites are more likely than the general population to have higher incidence and death statistics for certain types of cancer, largely due to lack of medical coverage, barriers to early detection and screening, unequal access to improvements in cancer treatment, and a combination of hazardous occupations and degraded living conditions where exposure to environmental toxins has intensified the risk of developing and decreased the chances of surviving cancer.[75] Discrepancies in survival are particularly evident at the intersections of race and gender: the highest death rate from cervical cancer is among African American women, and while white women have the highest incidence rate for breast cancer, African American women are most likely to die from the disease and experience—at a younger age—aggressive tumors that are poorly detected (due to unequal access to early screening and medical coverage) and less responsive to standard cancer treatments.[76] African American men have the highest incidence rate for prostate cancer and are more than twice as likely as white men to die of the disease.[77]

The affect of hope plays a specific role in obfuscating these deaths—and such obfuscation can itself lead to excess deaths, precisely because the causes of racialized and classed-based cancer incidence are not adequately addressed. In cancer culture, hope works to obscure the political character of the disease—for example, in the lack of attention directed toward cancer-causing toxicity and pollution and differential access to healthy environments, food choices, and the biomedical embrace. In this regard, there are "hope haves" and "hope have-nots." While the Patient Protection and Affordable Care Act was signed into law in 2010 to remedy health disparities and eradicate this "hope divide," universal health care access remains highly uneven, particularly in cancer-related care and health outcomes.[78] As the racial/ethnic and gender differences in the financial hardships of medical debt indicate, no amount of hoping for the biomedical cure for cancer will resolve the linkages between health status differences and other structural inequalities especially related to homeownership, insurance, environmental location and conditions, poverty, and so forth.[79]

The deployment of hope also eclipses the realities of the disease by refusing a space to address fear, precarity, uncertainty, and pain; for S. Lochlann Jain, "*that* politics and suffering is more easily black-boxed behind chipper wrapping paper."[80] The affect of hope is constructed as militantly positive and future oriented, and the disease can only be approached as something to be overcome, surmounted, or vanquished. This kind of hope is what is called on as the acceptable and, indeed, the only possible response to cancer diagnosis and treatment, because it is this kind of hope that facilitates the triumphant march onward—to more life. The problem here is obviously not hope in and of itself but the particular conventions of hope that are normalized within biocultures of cancer and the reality that only certain kinds of life can be affirmed and hoped for—positive, ongoing life. The affirmation of life, conditioned through the conventions of hope that we have analyzed, leaves little room to meditate on death or the collateral damage of living under the shadow of imminent death, and it renders invisible those individuals who can be said to "live out" the let-die component of biopolitics. The vulnerability of the subject with cancer does not, cannot, register. These are the *other* lives, ones that fail to achieve "life" as it is known in dominant knowledge systems and/or those lives abandoned, truncated, or elided in the social sphere.

In short, hope is not inherently "good," nor is the affirmation of life. Rather, hope, as it operates in the biomedical arena and broader social sphere in relation to cancer most specifically, has an ominous quality, with pernicious effects. Hope obscures the regulatory and political–economic nature of the affirmation of life and circumscribes social responsibility and ethics. It places the onus on the individual as an agent for life and fosters a limited approach to that life. In the context of these conventions of hope, precious few alternative expressions or tactics of hope and life in relation to cancer exist. Such alternative imaginings are generally overshadowed—or risk being deemed pathological—because of their failure to assemble and reflect acceptable responses to the disease. Despite this, we conclude with several key examples *that imagine hope otherwise.* These "hopeful" alternatives show how hope might be understood not as militant affirmation but as practices that attend to death and precarity through recognition of vulnerability. In these alternative imaginings, what is hoped for is more tangible, modest, and immediate than triumphant survival.

The Beautiful and Bald Movement, for instance, began a public campaign in 2011 to convince toy maker Mattel to mass-produce a bald Barbie doll called "Hope," "in support of children living with hair loss due to chemotherapy, alopecia, trichotillomania and other auto-immune diseases."[81] This demand for the Hope Barbie took the form of social-networking activism, operating primarily on Facebook, and has had overwhelming public support, with more than 135,000 fans as of March 2016.[82] A prototype of the doll that Mattel did produce sported a magnificent diamante-encrusted, black ball-gown, a pink stole, and a tiara on her proudly displayed bald head. Such a doll offers an alternative to the contemporary "makeover" imperative that compels cancer to be hidden through the maintenance of normative femininity, which is largely signified through hair, and instead actualizes the public display of cancer in its depiction of the harsh physical effects of treatments. Had it been released on the mass market, this doll could have potentially provided children with hope for other models of femininity. While still working within the commercial hope culture and representing dominant norms of female embodiment, Hope Barbie could have simultaneously subverted those norms by resignifying hair loss, reimagining beauty, and depicting a tantalizing drag or glam superhero version of Barbie—with cancer.[83] The possibility of such a doll, however, was resisted by Andrew Becker, director of media relations for the ACS, who stated that the Hope Barbie would "do more harm than good for kids and parents" and that children "could . . . end up being terrorized by the prospect of it [cancer] in a far outsized proportion to their realistic chances [of developing the disease]."[84] Hope Barbie, for Becker (and by extension the ACS), would lead to the evacuation of hope, presumably due to the realities that the doll would embody.

A second example of alternative imaginings of hope is at work in the organization called Hope Cancer Ministries (HCM).[85] This nonprofit, faith-based ministry provides practical care and assistance for patients, caregivers, and families living with cancer by offering services like transportation, meals, home handymen, housekeeping, and financial support for critical needs (for example, utility bills). These services attend to the day-to-day needs and the hard realities of those affected by cancer and its accompanying treatments when, for instance, the need for a ride to chemotherapy or childcare is often more immediate than hope for the cure. In the absence of a custodial state that might attend to the concerns of those living with illness, HCM presents a necessary safety net. It moves away from individualistic framings of hope and instead deploys faith in the service of a practical *community* of health. While such practices might be criticized for offering only a compromised hope that fails to address the social and political inadequacies of the health care system, ultimately, *hoping for help in the daily practice of living with and possibly dying of cancer* represents a revised vision of hope: as that which must be continually reoriented. In this sense, the hope offered by HCM dovetails with palliative care ideology and practice that, rather than reproducing the endless "hope through treatment" and "hope in the cure," faces death by focusing on caring—not curing—and giving credence to the possibility of dying well. By promoting nonhospitalized care at the end of life, palliative care and HCM provide the dying with hope for more quality time with loved ones, pain and symptom management, emotional or spiritual support in approaching death, and, ultimately, a good death.

Finally, Bob Carey's photographic series The Tutu Project gestures toward more modest and tentative forms of hope in relation to cancer culture—wherein, as Jain has stated, "hope and exceptionalism pervade . . .

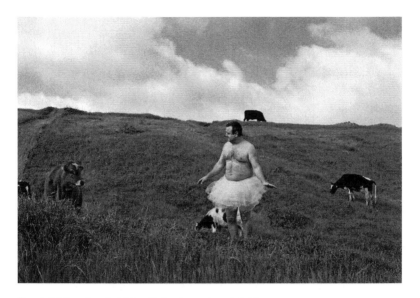

Figure 2. Bob Carey, Cows (2005), from The Tutu Project. Copyright Bob Carey.

like a shrill thread, everyone hanging on for dear life and yet still dangling."[86] In this whimsical set of images, Carey photographs himself in various locales—cornfields, barren hilltops, hanging on to a climbing wall, in the middle of a street in the snow—wearing only a scant pink tulle tutu. Inspired initially by Carey's wife's diagnosis of breast cancer, the project raises awareness and funds for breast cancer research and might be said to stage an implicit critique of dominant breast cancer conventions. A man wearing a pink tutu calls into question the feminization of breast cancer culture; a man frolicking, prancing, bounding, or standing as a diminutive figure in an unexpected landscape (a deserted subway station, a darkened parking lot, a cow paddock) conveys a playfulness that highlights the conservatism of cancer politics; and Carey's lone and near-naked body stands at odds with the mass spectacle of cancer in the broader public sphere. Through depicting Carey's lone figure, his face generally turned from the viewer, in often absurd locations and scenarios, these alternative renderings also introduce melancholy and vulnerability into the representation of cancer and thus push away hope as relentless optimism and the conviction to survive. Instead, hope emerges as a subtle, even solitary—though not an individualistic—subjunctive possibility and as a sharing of humor in times

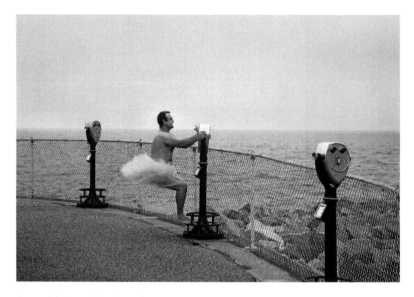

Figure 3. Bob Carey, Lookout *(2008), from* The Tutu Project. *Copyright Bob Carey.*

of distress and fear. As Carey has stated, "cancer has taught us that life is good, dealing with it can be hard, and sometimes the very best thing—no, the only thing—we can do to face another day is to laugh at ourselves, and share a laugh with others."[87] His articulations do not prioritize the commercialization of hope, thus enabling the politics of cancer to be foregrounded. They do not represent hope as unencumbered triumphalism but instead seek space for dealing with messiness, fragility, absurdity, and loss and attempt to foster creative and even playful forms of persistence. In one particular image, Carey stoops against a barbed-wire fence on what appears to be the deserted edges of a city. Rubbish gathered around the fence surrounds him, while a Goodyear blimp floats in the sky above. Such an image might be said to ironically juxtapose the concept of elevation and the vision of the horizon (and the hope for a good year?) with limits (the barbed-wire fence), abandonment, solitude, and the detritus of daily life. Hope, here, is a practice of "artful endurance."[88]

Taken together, these alternative articulations of hope still affirm life, but they do not necessarily frame that life as exclusive of death. Moreover, these other ways of hoping perform the difficult and often painful labor of persisting within the realities of cancer and the fear that can accompany it.

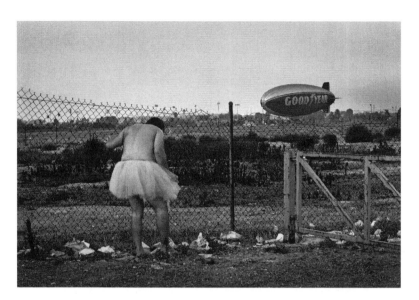

Figure 4. Bob Carey, Blimp (2008), from The Tutu Project. Copyright Bob Carey.

Instead of marshaling militant hope, these kinds of hope are fragile; they show forms of mourning, maintenance work, and humor. Rather than being predicated on future orientation, they focus on grappling with the present. Ultimately, these articulations might be said to operate as critiques of the dominant conventions of hope: they intervene into and redirect the ways that hope has come to operate and be deployed to govern populations, communities, and senses of self in relation to cancer. Here critique operates as "an instrument for those who fight, resist, and who refuse what is. . . . It is a challenge directed to what is."[89] It signals a refusal to be governed "like that and at that cost"[90] and advances *an incitement to hope otherwise.*

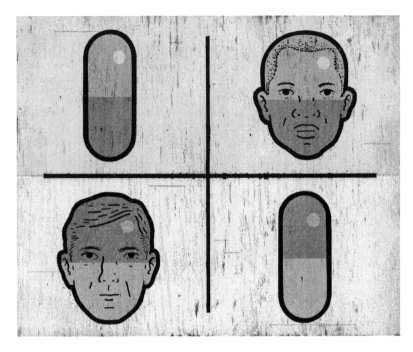

Figure 5. Copyright Dan Page c/o theispot.

2

Target

Race

> *Over time, providers who work with high utilizers are able to categorize patients into distinct groups ... [one of which is described as] "socially disintegrated," [those] who tend not to engage in self-care, have few family resources and display dependent personalities.*
>
> —Haydn Bush, "Health Care's Costliest 1%"

> *The student must ignore ... these extreme statements and seek to extract from a complicated mass of facts the tangible evidence of a social atmosphere surrounding Negroes, which differs from that surrounding most whites; of a different mental attitude, moral standard, and economic judgment shown toward Negroes than most other folk.*
>
> —W. E. B. Du Bois, *The Philadelphia Negro*

On August 1, 1896, W. E. B. Du Bois began a fifteen-month-long socio-logical study commissioned by the University of Pennsylvania, which was eventually published as *The Philadelphia Negro: A Social Study* (1899).[1] Widely recognized as the first great empirical book on black life in American society, Du Bois's study included an analysis of the health conditions of Philadelphia's black population and might be seen as part of a *race-specific biopolitics of health* within the biocultural sphere. The biopolitics of health, in its most general sense, refers to the administration of health that manages and standardizes the life of the population—to make the "biological citizens" of the nation live more.[2] What Du Bois makes clear in his study, however, is that the administration of the biological life of the population in the United States has been "cut" by racism and entrenched racial disparities.

Indeed, the first function of racism, Michel Foucault tells us, is "to fragment, to create caesuras within the biological continuum."[3] The "cut" of racism has meant that different segments of the population have been administered in distinct ways and, importantly, that white lives have been affirmed and made to live in ways that other lives have not. As Michael Dillon and Andrew W. Neal have argued, race functions as a marker that biopolitically adjudicates: race "does not only specify life's eligibilities for this or that good—it ultimately specifies whether or not a life is to be considered eligible for life as such."[4] Viewed through this lens, the differential governing or management of black subjects—Du Bois's focus—both often operates as a form of violence against the black body/subject and situates African Americans as separate from the wider population and the polis. Du Bois's investigation highlights that the city of Philadelphia—by way of commissioning this work—*sought to better manage and secure* what were seen as the potentially dangerous problems of the African American population.[5] It is in this way that the study operated as a race-specific bio-politics of health, wherein black life (and blackness itself) was articulated as an ontological problem (the infamous "Negro problem") to be studied, measured, and ultimately contained.[6] The political problem of black life was deemed the *product* of supposed inherent black difference—a difference that required regulation. Du Bois both refused and inverted this logic: re-framing the so-called Negro problem in terms of environmental factors and relentless historical disenfranchisement, he showed that African American problems regarding health were "largely a matter of the condition of living."[7] Ultimately, Du Bois insisted that, as a problem produced through social conditions, black health—or lack thereof—needed to be attended to and normalized in line with the cultivation of white subjects. We might say, then, that the Du Boisian study was a demand that the "cut" in the biopolitical fostering of life—along the color line—be remedied through a more affirmative focus on black health. For Du Bois, however, this would be achieved not through a focus on blackness as a "problem" but through addressing the manifold social factors that thwart black life.

Biomedical Targeting of Race

Contemporary biomedical technologies that target race seem to ameliorate the "cut" of systemic racism—by targeting supposedly race-specific health factors or directing health care toward particular spaces to alleviate health disparities.[8] We view these biomedical targeting technologies as part of broader biocultures of race-based health—an often-amorphous arena that encompasses efforts in (and relays between) the biological sciences, clinical medicine and public health, the pharmaceutical industry, and patient and community-based advocacy to address health and illness through the lens of race. In what follows, we consider two examples of biomedical targeting technologies and their biopolitical and disciplinary operations. First, we focus on BiDil, a pharmaceutical approved by the U.S. Food and Drug Administration (FDA) in 2005 and subsequently marketed as a race-specific drug for self-identified African Americans suffering from heart failure. Second, we turn to what is known as "medical hot-spotting," a practice that began in Camden, New Jersey, in 2007 and that uses GIS technologies and spatial profiling to identify populations that are medically vulnerable ("health care's costliest 1%") to provide preemptive care at home and lower hospital admissions and health care costs. These targeting technologies—or operations—are deployed ostensibly to affirm life within biocultures of race-based health: they are said to redress past forms of biomedical neglect and enable the tailoring of biomedical intervention into vulnerable communities, and they are advocated as the means through which to foster the health of those populations—through attention, through targeting. Such forms of redress and attention might be understood, then, as the attempt to practice—and actualize—a different racial future, precisely through attending to inequities in the present.

However, targeted health interventions may in effect signal inequitable and endangering forms of biomedical administration.[9] We advance this more cautionary view through three foundational claims. First, regardless of the motivations for biomedical targeting—that is, the will to attend to minority health—the operation of race-specific biomedical targeting is *structured through dominant epistemologies of race* that position nonwhites as Other to the normative Human. More than racist actions or the architecture of racial discrimination, this form of knowledge designates nonwhite subjects as the constitutive outside of the normative world. Not only has this dominant epistemology of race shaped the racial past in the United States but it also curtails the present and future of nonwhite life. Specifically in relation to black subjects—who live in a paradigm that binds blackness and death together—it is a form of knowledge that positions the black subject *outside* of the category Human.[10] This positioning stems from liberal humanist thought and is constitutive of Western modernity.[11] Such expulsion of black lives from the normative position Human is undeniable, "given the histories of slavery, colonialism, segregation, lynching," and the ongoing daily imperiling of black lives through police brutality and mass incarceration.[12] That biomedical targeting is structured through such epistemologies of race is evident in the way it reinstitutes racial difference and separation and, as we will show, stages an additional form of violence by actually expelling blacks from the possibility of optimal health. Black lives have been consistently imperiled in and through the biomedical encounter, in the form of lack of access to care and health insurance, inequities in caregiving, and the medical abuse of black bodies, from grave robbing for medical experimentation to the Tuskegee Syphilis Experiments and the appropriation of the Henrietta Lacks cell line.[13] Anti-black racism continues to thwart black life and futurity through biomedical targeting operations that subject African Americans to what Du Bois named as a "social atmosphere . . . which differs from that surrounding whites."[14] Race-based targeting efforts that are aimed at redressing health inequities actually recursively secure this dominant epistemology of racial Otherness by refusing to acknowledge its structuring logic, thus equating blackness with inevitable vulnerability, risk, threat, and premature death.[15] Importantly, while we focus mainly on blackness in this chapter (because citizenship/subjectivity has been constituted in relation to African Americans so differently to other racial groups in the United States), the medical apartheid set up through race-based targeting can and does extend to capture other racialized groups. This becomes particularly clear in our analysis of medical hot-spotting, where we see Latinx and native communities enfolded within—subjected to—such differential governing.[16]

Second, and related to our first point, these biomedical targeting operations *extract the conditions of minority health and illness* from the broader contexts of structural racism. By this, we mean that biomedical targeting generally fails to recognize the social conditions in which poor health emerges and how poor health, institutional racism, and the epistemology of racial Otherness are ontologically enmeshed. Indeed, the targeting of racialized populations—specifically through the two cases we explore here—does not simply direct resources to underserved groups. Instead, in such operations, race is *objectified* as that to be targeted, meaning that race itself is thus *not undone*: that is, race as a stratifying mechanism that orders the social is not called into question. Both BiDil and medical hot-spotting demarcate populations, with supposedly distinct bodies, and name them as a political problem in need of specific health governance; nonwhite bodies and racialized spaces are targeted in order to manage the life of the population. Accordingly, BiDil might be seen to ontologize blackness as a corporeal truth for market accumulation, while medical hot-spotting can be said to spatially ontologize structural racism to secure cost efficiencies of the health care system. BiDil is predicated on financial extraction; medical hot-spotting is predicated on threat containment.

These biomedical targeting technologies reveal how health interventions within contemporary biocultures of race-based health do not necessarily support or achieve a better future for underserved minority populations. Instead, they advance an epistemological violence by concentrating the "problem" of racialized life in the United States at the scales of (1) the racialized body (BiDil) and (2) space (hot spots), which both become objects of ever more heightened administration, financial exploitation, and securitization. BiDil positions African Americans as "problem bodies" that must take on responsibility for their own racialized embodied risk through the act of buying and consuming race-based medicine; here racial governance of health operates through the black responsibilization of risk. Medical hot-spotting tracks, maps, and fixes high-cost health care users in "problem spaces" that are positioned outside of the rest of the populace; hot-spotting locates and reifies the structural position of racial Otherness in space for the purposes of surveillance, anticipation of risk, and containment.

Third, contemporary biomedical targeting technologies are an endangering form of health administration *exacerbated by the logics of neoliberalism.* Under neoliberal conditions, populations previously excluded from the vital politics of the nation are now ostensibly being addressed. However, the two biomedical targeting technologies that we explore reveal a *predatory power* to demarcate race for purposes spanning financial extraction to threat containment (as we note earlier)—even as such "targeting" is advocated as the means for addressing the embodied and spatial effects of racial inequality. In neoliberal times, the color line no longer operates as a clear and obvious modality of exclusion, as Du Bois would have it.[17] The neoliberal biopolitics of health increasingly emphasizes *customizing* health, the body, and life itself through biomedical practices.[18] Our two case studies reveal how customizing health seems to be an operation of inclusion (directly or indirectly by race) within dominant biocultures of race-based health: BiDil is a customized drug that attends to black health; it targets African Americans supposedly to extend life. Medical hot-spotting is also a form of customization through care delivery: it locates "problem spaces"—where high utilizers of health care are located—to direct resources and generate efficiencies in health provisions. "Customizing" works in the first case through "color awareness" and marketing within biomedicine and the pharmaceutical industry (i.e., the racialized spectacle of the body) and

paradoxically, in the second, through invisibilizing race at the level of loca-
tion/space according to the so-called color-blind agency of the free market
and cost–benefit analysis.[19] While both targeting technologies may attempt
to alleviate racial health disparities, they simultaneously augment racial
difference and exacerbate racial inequalities—*but they do so in very different ways*: thus emphasizing the importance of tracing out the empirically
distinct means through which each technology resecures the epistemology
of racial Otherness. BiDil highlights the neoliberal refusal to acknowledge the social production of risk by casting health as an individual—not
social—enterprise. Medical hot-spotting disavows the historical and spatial
processes of racial formation that structure the present and simultaneously
shows that certain (racialized) subjects are positioned—in advance—as risk
failures within the paradoxically "race-neutral future" of the nation. To
begin exploring these ideas, we turn to the case of BiDil, the oft-disputed
first pharmaceutical with a race-specific indication.

Race Drugs: BiDil and Customizing Health "For Blacks Only"

On June 24, 2005, the *New York Times* announced that "the Food and
Drug Administration took a controversial step toward a new frontier of
personalized medicine yesterday, approving the first drug ever intended
for one racial group, African Americans."[20] This new pharmaceutical,
marketed as BiDil, targeted racial health and promised to both revolu-
tionize biomedical attention to racial disparities and pave the way toward
pharmacogenomics—where drugs and drug combinations will be optimized for each individual's unique genetic makeup.[21] According to the
pharmaceutical company NitroMed (then owner of the patented drug),
BiDil is "for use in addition to routine medicines to treat heart failure in
African American patients, to extend life, improve heart failure symptoms,
and help heart failure patients stay out of the hospital longer."[22]

BiDil did not begin as a race-specific drug but, rather, became one
through what Jonathan Kahn has called "a complex array of legal, commercial, and medical circumstances that transformed the drug's identity."[23]
The clinical trial that finally led to BiDil's approval, the African-American
Heart Failure Trial (A-HeFT),[24] was conducted after many years of trying to
get the drug off the ground: this trial enrolled *only* black patients, and NitroMed sought a race-specific approval because that indication had a longer
remaining patent life.[25] A-HeFT compared standard-of-care treatment plus

placebo with standard-of-care treatment plus BiDil, a new combination of two existing generic drugs, hydralazine hydrochloride and isosorbide dinitrate. While the A-HeFT trial ended early—having convincingly proved that BiDil was beneficial for lowering the risk of death—it did not compare different racial groups and thus the trial did not actually prove race-specific efficacy. The FDA, however, cleared BiDil as *only for use in black patients.*[26]

Essentially, BiDil identifies, names, localizes, and depicts African Americans as a distinct group—that can be clearly demarcated—in order to make that group into an accessible "object" for the drug's development, approval, marketing, and consumption. Within the broad biocultural arena, BiDil was identified as a necessary "good." Organizations such as the Association of Black Cardiologists recognized BiDil as a means to address the specific health needs of African Americans and as a remedy for enduring health disparities to save black lives. The NAACP, too, backed the race-based drug by prioritizing the immediate needs of black individuals having access to medicines that would work—rather than focusing on the risks of the drug's racialized designation. At the same time, however, many were wary of racial profiling in medicine and its associated risks and the way BiDil might further pathologize risk within the black body.

This latter line of thought directs attention to one of the key problematics of BiDil as an example of race-based biomedical targeting in neoliberal times: it reaffirms and ontologizes racial difference in the space of the body as a biological truth—*at the genetic level.* As Kahn has argued, "underlying the [BiDil] trial design is a race-specific patent that is premised on a genetic conception of race."[27] The FDA approval for BiDil was also ultimately predicated on this idea, as the organization gave its (and thus the state's) imprimatur to the claim that African Americans had a different—and implicitly substandard[28]—physiology of the heart, attributable to some unknown but inherent biological factor.[29] While the participants in the A-HeFT trial (that led to the FDA approval) were not genetically tested, "race" was used as a marker and a descriptor—a proxy—for genetics in the case of BiDil.[30] Such a move problematically means that people with radically varying genetic realities are homogenized under the racial descriptor "African American." It assumes that racial groups are biologically distinct (that there are clear lines between different races) and that African Americans represent a unitary racial group; it suggests that race itself is biological rather than a social category.[31] As Troy Duster has poignantly argued, however, the issue of black heart failure "was not biological or genetic in origin, but biological in effect due to stress-related outcomes of reduced access to valued social goods, such as employment, promotion, housing stock, etc. The *effect* was biological, not the origins."[32]

There is no denying that BiDil reduces heart failure. It is not clear, however, that it operates in a racially specific way. The deployment of BiDil as a "solution" to black ill health elides how the workings of anti-black racism *register* at the level of biology, as Duster suggests, and directs resources—a pill—at the *effects* of anti-black racism. This directing of resources at effects rather than causes reaffirms the correlation between biologically based notions of blackness and risk. Biomedical targeting, then, as in the case of BiDil, abstracts bodies from material space (and history) and naturalizes the historical conditioning of the black body as separate from template (white) "Human embodiment." Indeed, BiDil might be viewed as a reinstantiation of the epistemology of racial Otherness in that the black body itself is viewed as the "problem" that needs a separate form of biopolitical administration. Ironically, then, while the pill might be seen as a way to decondition the historical accumulation of anti-black racism, it actually augments its operation.

The second key problematic highlighted in the case of BiDil is that such targeting can financialize supposed racial difference (and life itself) through customization and *render this difference a market opportunity.* Indeed, race—and specifically the supposed racial difference of African Americans—became the means through which to overturn the previous FDA rejection of BiDil and to create a niche market, rendering the black body a biocommodity[33] or what Jonathan Inda has called a locus of "vital value."[34] What we see, then, is that nonwhite consumers represent an emerging growth market to be targeted by drug manufacturers precisely because of the high incidence rates of certain diseases *within* minority communities: while these diseases are themselves often caused by or exacerbated through operations of past and present biopolitical neglect, the biological effects of racial injustice *become the basis* for a profit-making enterprise.[35]

This BiDil marketing opportunity—located in the suffering black body—was spectacularly financialized: there was an estimated market of 750,000 black Americans out of a total 5 million people with heart disease who might benefit from the pill, and Wall Street analysts predicted "annual sales of US$500 million, even $1 billion by 2010."[36] Stock prices promised to be equally impressive, and in the lead-up to the FDA approval, BiDil stock crested at $29 per share.[37] The part of the revenue that would stem from sales of the drug was to be secured through BiDil's pricing structure: each pill cost $1.80, and patients would be required to take six pills per day. Had the drug been successful (ultimately, it was not), a regimen of BiDil would cost $10.80 per day and $3,942 per year, making the drug between four and seven times more expensive than the combined price for the generic drugs out of which it was made.[38] Thus, despite the fact that BiDil ostensibly represented the fostering of life—of African Americans and, potentially, all patients—it did not necessarily support a better future for African Americans. If physicians were encouraged to prescribe this drug (to the exclusion of other therapies) because of its racial indication, yet acquiring it was financially prohibitive, then African Americans were perversely expelled from the opportunity to attain optimal health. BiDil clearly represented an exploitative accumulation strategy enabled through customization, one that would make money from black suffering. BiDil exemplifies how neoliberal race-specific biopolitics operates through racialized *bioeconomics*—the economic exploitation of the unequal conditions of racial life. It reveals an economic calculus that profits from the continuation of racialized ill health, which, ironically, the drug was meant to alleviate.

The third problematic of race-based biomedical targeting in the case of BiDil is that personalized care was implicitly framed as only achievable through the black responsibilization of health and risk. As Nikolas Rose has noted more generally, the contemporary biocitizen is called on to "partake of the ethic of active citizenship that has taken shape in advanced liberal democracies."[39] The idea—and attendant ethic—of active citizenship increasingly encourages people to self-care as a *biological responsibility*. Precisely because BiDil was approved and marketed as a heart failure therapy "for African Americans," it presented an opportunity—and a call—for black subjects to attend to their health by way of consuming the drug. Two key factors should be noted here. To attend to health—to assume this responsibility—required that a new form of biosociality be inaugurated: a further collective identification of people of African descent, predicated now on supposed genetic sameness.[40] The racial indication for BiDil required that blacks claim race as a biological truth, target themselves on the basis of this supposed truth, and govern themselves accordingly to fulfill the call to attend to health. Essentially, black subjects were entreated to "consume blackness" through using a designer black drug that, as we have outlined, was itself predicated on reductive and biologically essentialist ideas of race.[41]

Additionally, the "problem" of black health would be borne by the affected *individuals*. This individual responsibility for health is in line with
neoliberal logics and practices more generally that have seen the devolution
of state powers and collective securitization by the state and a shift toward
the privatized and individualized government of risk. In the case of BiDil,
it is evident that black health was cast as a biological factor for which African Americans need to be responsible—rather than a social product for
which there might be a general social responsibility. The individualization
of health can also be seen in the fact that the financial burden of BiDil
would not be shared: Medicaid did not always cover the drug or states did
not require Medicare plans to include it, and private insurance companies
also denied coverage.[42] Ultimately, then, the drug was put out of reach for
the majority of those people it purported to help. This operation suggests
a continuation of state and now privatized disinterest in African American
health. The case of BiDil can be seen as exposing African Americans to a
neoliberal expulsion from health: a drug that was ostensibly made to affirm
black life was available but not *made* available.[43] The irony is that such lack
of availability, coupled with poor patient demand and the unwillingness of
doctors to prescribe the drug, contributed to BiDil's failure to secure the
projected revenue and led to its eventual demise.[44]

Inarguably, BiDil can be viewed as a drug that offered (and continues
to offer) the potential to affirm black lives, not by virtue of the racial speci-
fication, but by the simple fact that the drug has been shown to work. As
Inda has powerfully argued, BiDil represents a way of realizing vital rights
for black lives, a means to attend to racial health disparities, and a vehicle
through which to materialize hope in communities affected by an excess
burden of illness.[45] But BiDil also problematically reifies anti-black racism
in biomedicine and society more broadly and shows that drug companies
can and have profited at the expense of the suffering black body. The meanings presented in the case of BiDil are inherently polarized and, indeed,
contradictory, and it is this slippage—between positive and negative aspects
of the drug—that leads Anne Pollock to characterize BiDil as a pharmakon,
that is, as having "the capacity to be beneficial and detrimental *to the same
person at the same time.*"[46] Ultimately, however, the ontologizing of black
health in the space (and as the property) of the black body resecures the
ideas both that black corporeality itself is the "problem" and that blackness
equates with risk, suggesting that, by and large, the detrimental aspects of
the drug actually overwhelm the beneficial.

Locating the 1 Percent: Medical Hot-Spotting and Racialized Biosecurity

The contradictions and racialized hazards of biomedical targeting within contemporary biocultures of race-based health are further illustrated in our second case study, on medical hot-spotting. *Medical hot-spotting* refers to "a problem-solving technique that targets the most expensive problems or in-need people by allocating resources to specific problem areas as revealed by the data."[47] It endeavors to reorganize health governance according to the economic logic of cost efficiency by targeting populations that are "high utilizers"—that incur high costs—in the U.S. health care system.[48] The practice began in Camden, New Jersey, an economically depressed community across the Delaware River from Philadelphia. Following the collapse of its industrial base and decades of disinvestment, Camden effectively became a container of poverty within a deeply racialized region, with declining interior infrastructure and minimal access to outlying areas where services were being elevated and communities cultivated.[49] The city of Camden today hosts a slew of toxic industries, from incinerators that burn Philadelphia's trash to pharmaceuticals manufacturing. The city's housing and infrastructure are largely unsafe or abandoned, and the population (~77,000) is per capita one of the poorest in the nation.[50] In 2006—just prior to the adoption of medical hot-spotting—the median household income in Camden City was $18,007, the lowest of all U.S. communities with populations over 65,000, and 52 percent of the city's residents lived in poverty.[51] These figures become particularly telling in light of the racial demographics of the city: according to the 2010 census, half of the city's residents were black or African American, and more than a third of the residents were "Latino or Hispanic."[52] Widespread industrial contamination, poverty, and escalated violent crime all have contributed to a dire public health problem in Camden. With 29.5 percent of the population unable to afford prescription drugs, the city's residents clearly experience disproportionate levels of ill health.[53]

The innovations of medical hot-spotting emerged in this racialized context as a means to lower exorbitant health care spending on the medically indigent by coordinating intensive outpatient care for complex high-needs patients.[54] The practice involves locating costly users of the health care system and targeting them for more effective, preemptive care to cut down on the number of medical crises requiring expensive treatments and rehospitalizations. To achieve this, medical hot-spotting applies policing strategies to health care, namely, the methods of tracking and mapping crime statistics to direct police to "hot spots" of criminal activity.[55] The medical application of this police technology uses medical data to identify populations that are high utilizers or "super-users" of the health care system, that is, patients who use health care resources at abnormally high rates. Medical hot-spotting in Camden revealed that 1 percent of patients were driving 30 percent of medical costs and that people with the highest medical costs and the greatest number of emergency room visits were usually receiving the worst care.[56] One single public housing development was alone responsible for $12 million in health care costs from 2002 to 2008.[57] High utilizers of health care in Camden visited overburdened local clinics; they were uninsured or otherwise remiss about seeing a primary care doctor for preventive care, were on welfare and otherwise poor, and were purportedly making detrimental lifestyle choices with little capacity for change.[58] By targeting these concentrated zones of high utilizers through spatial data analysis, medical hot-spotting seeks to organize and tailor care management through numerous techniques that restructure the organization, delivery, accountability, and doctor–patient relations of health care, from interdisciplinary teamwork to house calls and behavioral modification techniques (focused on an individual patient for up to six months).[59] A promising aspect of medical hot-spotting, then, is its potential to alleviate health inequities, through stabilizing both the medical conditions *and* social environment of patients as a means to health. This might entail health and wellness promotion and psychosocial counseling, helping patients apply for government assistance programs, securing better housing or temporary shelter, and adapting to home life after hospital discharge.[60]

From its Camden origins, medical hot-spotting has gained traction across the health care system. Similar practices are now at work in places such as Trenton, Newark, West Philadelphia, York, Scranton, Allentown, the Bronx and Queens, Atlantic City, Boston, Anchorage, Chicago, Seattle, and Las Vegas.[61] Such health care reforms and experimentations are needed *social projects,* which, we argue, are always *inherently racial projects.*[62] Indeed, the well-documented institutional racism of biomedicine and persistent forms of structural racism that underpin U.S. society and produce differential vulnerabilities to illness and disease are part of what universal access to health care endeavors to address and even rectify.[63] Yet "race" remains topically out of bounds in discussions about medical hot-spotting. Our contribution, then, is to consider the racialized operations and potentially inequitable and endangering effects of medical hot-spotting as a relatively new practice of targeted health interventions. While BiDil might be said to ontologize blackness as a *corporeal* truth for market accumulation, the neoliberal logics and spatial technologies of medical hot-spotting work to *ontologize racialized spaces*—they ontologize structural racism *as space,* as transparent/self-evident, race-neutral, dehistoricized, undialectical space. Regardless of the intentions behind medical hot-spotting, it potentially supports intensified racial dominance under the auspices of improved health administration and biosecurity. We explore here three developments on the horizon of U.S. health care reform that rationalize the epistemology of racial Otherness through intensifying forms of monitoring and containing costs. Such speculative analysis is timely given the mounting popularity of medical hot-spotting under the banner "when treating patients like criminals make sense."[64]

First, medical hot-spotting mobilizes a national imagination of scarce health care dollars and advances a world defined by a grid of relationships of cost that fuels racial enmities.[65] The abstraction of this cost grid disregards the "richness" of space—the social–spatial relationships that contribute to high-cost usage of health care—and it circumscribes subjectivity within the market. Managing medical care for cost containment disregards the structural reasons for ill health by giving epistemological primacy to cost relations.[66] There are countless examples of this circulating in the media: "there's a small segment that is burning through 20 percent of our society's wealth at a massive rate" or "because U.S. hospitals give billions of uncompensated care to the uninsured and under-insured each year, they pass costs along to insured users."[67] In the context of austerity policies and widespread panic about the overtaxed U.S. health care system, "cost efficiency" amplifies a racist antagonism between those who are worthy of scarce resources—an imagined community of deserving Americans, that is, white, suburban, healthy families—set against the despicable, leeching "high utilizers," a category that serves as a proxy for racialized others. The call to locate the super-user 1 percent marshals racism via the powerful rhetoric of statistics and unfair burden. We may see "high utilizer" join "welfare queen" and "gangbanger" in the pantheon of demonized subjects for "endangering our national health care budget and the health of worthy citizens who are not bringing health problems on themselves."[68]

Medical hot-spotting, then, easily supports the idea that hot spots are a threat to the nation and, by locating them, facilitates the transfer of blame and *placement of responsibility* on those who are already disadvantaged and disenfranchised, that is, those who inhabit these spaces. The super-user is identified and "found" through hot spot delineation, where the inhabitants-as-threat inhabit the space-as-threat, and vice versa. This is particularly deleterious to African Americans, who have received significantly less adequate care than white Americans because of a host of financial, organizational, and social barriers.[69] The historically accumulated suffering of the black body has meant that African Americans are at increased risk for acute and chronic diseases, epidemics like HIV/AIDS, and mental illness.[70] But disease burden and disparities in health exist across a range of racial and ethnic groups in the United States. For example, Latinx populations as a whole experience higher rates of diabetes, HIV infection, tuberculosis, cervical cancer, stomach cancer, liver cancer, and liver disease than whites.[71] In American Indian and Alaska Native adults, the age-adjusted death rate far exceeds that of the general population—by almost 40 percent—and deaths due to chronic liver disease and cirrhosis, tuberculosis, pneumonia and influenza, and heart disease also exceed those of the general population.[72] Health disparities also exist within the Asian American and Pacific Islander communities: Asian Americans experience the highest rates of any racial or ethnic group for liver, uterine, cervical, and stomach cancer;[73] Asian Americans and Pacific Islanders have greater incidence rates of tuberculosis and hepatitis B than any other racial or ethnic group; and Asian Americans experience higher rates of diabetes than whites.[74] The risks of racialized life in America are eclipsed, however, by operations that stratify the population and *justify* the harmful impacts of neoliberalization experienced disproportionately within certain minority communities.[75] Targeting the 1 percent of the U.S. health care system enacts a deeply structural logic of racism, equating racial difference with the antithesis of the ideal neoliberal citizen—as inherently vulnerable, risky, wasteful; as unable to be self-sufficient or healthy; and as a burden to the nation.

Second, medical hot-spotting promotes *self-care* in the absence of social welfare and thus contributes to a feedback loop of racial domination. Lack of health is attributed to personal failure rather than the structural positioning of black and brown subjects outside of the populace to be fostered, and the aggregation of these failures is mapped in space for the purposes of surveillance, anticipation of risk, and containment.[76] While autonomy and empowerment to make oneself be healthy are laudable goals, the neoliberal imperative to "self-care" undercuts the promise of *social* reform by enlisting the nation's costliest health care consumers to participate in preventive care—a process that relegates racially coded economic, social-environmental disadvantage to the private and personal spheres.[77] Neoliberal self-care asserts that *individuals* are solely in charge of their health and should *adjust their behavior* to achieve optimal health; individuals who fail to do so are "bad," deviant, or even pathological subjects, despite any structural issues that might preclude good health. Under neoliberal logics, minorities are enlisted to self-care—to participate as consumers of preventive care—yet any inability to do so is relegated to a private issue or racially grouped failure within a supposedly color-blind meritocracy enabled by the free market.[78] Thus, medical hot-spotting potentially resecures the epistemology of racial Otherness through requiring racialized subjects to take on self-responsibility as if it were race transcendent.

The practice seeks to intervene in the daily care of three categories of patients—the mentally ill, the medically fragile elderly, and patients who are described as "socially disintegrated," that is, "those who tend not to engage in self-care, have few family resources and display dependent personalities."[79] The category of "socially disintegrated" seemingly offers an opportunity to examine the race-specific biopolitics of health—how poor health, institutional racism, and the epistemology of racial Otherness are ontologically enmeshed. Anecdotal evidence and a short documentary about medical hot-spotting demonstrate that medical hot-spotting *does attempt* to expand health care into social, environmental arenas and to cultivate social infrastructure and stability through caregiving.[80] Such efforts, however, are undermined by the behaviorist emphasis, which medicalizes urban marginality. The sorting out of the so-called socially disintegrated—those who fail at/to self-care—from productive citizens allows for race to be understood as a marker of risky or dysfunctional social behaviors rather than an indicator of racialized knowledges and experiences that make one more vulnerable.[81] Medical hot-spotting signals a shift in health governance toward potentially more aggressive in/voluntary programs that target individual behavior and mandate personal responsibility, as the state is withdrawing institutional supports that are necessary to shoulder illness, unemployment, indigence, and so forth.[82] The practice could progress in the direction of racially sorting and segmenting health care to support *moralizing behavioral workfare* in the context of austerity and corporatized health care.

Third, medical hot-spotting risks spatially ontologizing historical geographies of racial domination—urban renewal, redlining in housing and mortgage industries, environmental racism—as simply geodemographic "facts" on a map. From crime mapping and policing, medical hot-spotting borrowed technologies (namely, CompStat) that collect and use spatial data to model, monitor, and control criminal behaviors. First instituted by then New York City Police Commissioner William Bratton in the mid-1990s, crime hot-spotting generates digital cartographic representations of high-crime areas by linking statistical information, such as crime type and occurrence, with zip code and neighborhood.[83] Police are then able to target anticipated high-crime spaces by spatially customizing surveillance and control.[84] Similarly, medical hot-spotting integrates GIS data and demographic techniques that target problem spaces and populations through spatial profiling.[85] Such geosurveillance is the logical outcome of the militarized interpretation of residents as risk factors that need to be logged, mapped, and understood in a calculative statistical manner. Medical hot-spotting secures target fields of information, spatial data, and geographical identification of high-risk people and spaces *for the purposes of biosecurity,* that is, managing health for the optimization of the population.[86] The auditing process—the geographical processing of medical metadata—generates a racially stratified datascape of expectations that basically reproduces "what we already know." The spatial ontology at work in this targeting operation stipulates that where you are reveals who you are, as collected, assessed, and defined by marketers, governments, the police, or clinics.[87] Racialized spaces and bodies become ontologized as knowable, measurable geotags and data of a population—even when medical hot-spotting does not explicitly involve racial profiling. In other words, medical hot-spotting *ontologizes structural racism in/as space.*

Medical hot-spotting's application of GIS demonstrates a political rationality that calls forth surveillant uses of technology in the observation of spaces and populations, transforming governing into a field of perception.[88] The geosurveillant technologies that inform medical hot-spotting arguably *mobilize the ghetto as a preemptive way of seeing,* of knowing-as-containing.[89] Thus, establishing medical hot spots may serve as a teleological spatial containment technique for the management of poverty and marginality.[90] Targeting the medically indigent 1 percent could result in "coordinated care camps" that punitively quarantine racialized segments of the population by restricting access to specialized medicine and experts. Stricter definitions of medical necessity may be instituted within hot spots to decrease opportunities to receive a particular test or treatment (a twisted reversal of current profit-seeking methods that overprescribe to the poor, such as ordering unnecessary tests or visits). Basically, medical hot-spotting allows for—even rationalizes—racially segmented care by drawing out and further entrenching social borders and spatial segregations. In other words, minority communities might experience medical hot-spotting as an intensified form of *medical redlining,* that is, "spatially customized care" as a means to ration medical resources and health care. Given the twin neoliberal imperatives of cost containment and self-care, it is not a stretch to see medical hot-spotting even develop into a *remote-sensored care delivery system* that somatically surveils the high utilizers of health care through cost-saving home monitoring, informatizes corporeal systems to mine data, and positions bodies as nodes within a network of physiological, behavioral, and locational data connected to command centers.[91] The geosurveillant technologies of medical hot-spotting reveal that health promotion and disease prevention involve increasingly militarized preemption, concentrated in preknown spaces of failure as analytic objects that can be surveilled at a distance.[92] Whether through self-responsibilization of risk or ontologizing structural racism in space, medical hot-spotting reveals the future of a race-specific biopolitics of health that rationalizes and defends *racialized biosecurity as race-neutral technology.*[93]

Abolitionist Biomedicine: Refusing *This* World

The Du Boisian vision of alleviating the racial "cut" in the governance of life has yet to be realized. In the era of neoliberal biopolitics, minority lives are imperiled in the very same moment that life is ostensibly affirmed. Biomedical targeting technologies are predicated on the seemingly laudable pursuit of attending to vulnerable populations and alleviating racial disparities of health. These technologies potentially address specific conditions of racial inequality, in accord with Du Bois's call to attend to the color line. In the contemporary era, race-based pharmaceuticals and medical hot-spotting bring underserved subjects into the fold of the vital politics of life through customizing care at different scales of existence—the individual body and the environment of certain populations. Yet, in doing so, as we have shown, these practices continue to ontologize those bodies and spaces as *a problem.* Thus, although they may not explicitly fortify the color line in the Du Boisian sense, they more ominously resecure racial division through the supposed fostering of life. The targeting of specific bodies or spaces extracts them from broader relations of structural racism and customizes medical resources in ways that objectify race or racialized space as that which should be secured against. Ultimately, such biomedical targeting recursively protects the reality that health optimization is an exclusionary project.

Our main intervention has been to examine the epistemological underpinnings of race-based health initiatives. Our two examples of BiDil and medical hot-spotting show that biomedical targeting anticipates risk and failure and performs death-expectant interventions that ultimately expel racial minorities from optimal health—but do so in different ways. BiDil extols black responsibility of risk, enlisting African Americans in self-care for lived and embodied conditions of anti-black racism—that is, for violence against blacks and for historically accumulated disadvantage and ill health that result from the positioning of African Americans outside of the category of Human. Medical hot-spotting further demonstrates the enduring workings of the epistemology of racial Otherness—through identifying "problem spaces" inhabited by "problem bodies." The practice orchestrates violence through spatial abstraction and data-based mapping operations that contain and surveil race as a threat, and, like BiDil, it calls for individualized responsibility. In short, such targeting fails to cultivate nonwhite futures and, instead, ontologically secures *minority status as nonfuturity.*

Futurity lies at the heart of biopolitical governance and practices, which intervene into life not only to control but also to *improve* the prospects of the population. In a Foucauldian understanding, biopolitics exerts a positive influence over life "that endeavors to administer, optimize, and multiply it, subjecting it to precise controls and comprehensive regulations."[94] Yet, if health, as we have shown, is an exclusionary achievement, it seems imperative to work to abolish race as an operation that biopolitically adjudicates. To this end, biomedical efforts that seek to organize reparative justice must work *against* reestablishing race as an ontology *at the very same moment* that we labor toward alleviating those very real social disparities predicated on race.[95] As such, a just politics would need to address race (and ethnicity) as the basis for health. Essentially, such a politics would *refuse this world,* precisely because it is structured through dominant epistemologies of race and "looks like no future at all."[96]

There is a strong history of these kinds of abolitionist medical efforts in the United States. For instance, President Johnson's "unconditional war on poverty" in the 1960s saw the establishment of the Office of Economic Opportunity, which funded the earliest form of community health centers in the United States. Such centers not only delivered face-to-face medical care to minority and poor individuals but also addressed the causes of poverty and the social etiologies of disease—looking to improve the social and environmental determinants of health: "they repaired old housing, built clean water and sanitary systems, organized food cooperatives, cleaned up environmental threats, created local transportation systems, developed potent community organizations, and—most important—trained and hired local residents as health workers at multiple levels, and opened pathways to professional education."[97]

In the 1970s, the Black Panther Party also advanced a range of health activism projects, based on their understanding of the links between race, economic disparities, and poor health. As part of their strategy to expand services in underserved communities, they operated numerous health clinics across the country—addressing health concerns in black communities, such as screening for sickle cell anemia. They also developed "survival programs" that pursued what Alondra Nelson has called "medical self-defense." The Free Breakfast for Children program fed more than twenty thousand children every week, with the aim of maximizing health. They offered community classes in economics, first aid, and self-defense; developed programs that provided drug and alcohol rehabilitation; supplied groceries and clothing to those in need; and organized escorts and advocates for seniors to attend medical appointments.[98] More than this, however, the Black Panther Party called for free health care for *all* black and oppressed peoples, highlighting the linkages between poverty and medical marginality regardless of race. In their revised 1972 Ten Points Program (the Panther Party platform for action), "health" was formally added as point 6—and reflected this commitment to health activism across racial lines:

We believe that the government must provide, free of charge, for the people, health facilities which will not only treat our illnesses, most of which have come about as a result of our oppression, but which will also develop preventative medical programs to guarantee our future survival. We believe that mass health education and research programs must be developed to give Black and oppressed people access to advanced scientific and medical information, so we may provide ourselves with proper medical attention and care.[99]

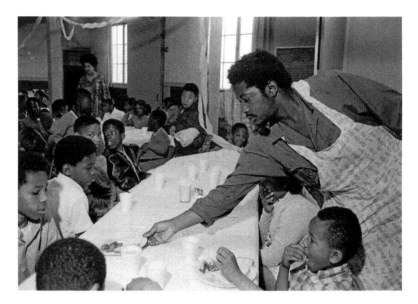

Figure 6. Charles Bursey hands a plate of food to a child seated at the Black Panthers' Free Breakfast program. Courtesy of Special Collections, University Library, University of California Santa Cruz, Pirkle Jones Photographs and Papers.

These historical examples highlight as much about what will be needed in the future as they reveal about the past.

Clearly the challenge continues, as evidenced by continued health disparities based on race, ethnicity, and poverty. The largest health gap is still race-based, between blacks and whites, in the United States. Black Lives Matter organizing and the practice of medical die-ins (part of the broader Black Lives Matter movement) have recently sought to address these enduring realities.[100] In response to the preemptive violence aimed at black individuals—and the long historical precedence of coercive force under which black people have been prefigured as threats in the United States—the multisited Black Lives Matter movement calls out and refuses the foundational logics of race, which only recognize and privilege white life and which position blacks as a population against which society must be defended. This refusal is enacted through the naming of a project *not yet realized*: that black lives matter.[101] The chant calls on people to repudiate the lethal conditions of living out the biopolitical cut of race in America—of no future for black lives—by asserting what biopolitical futurity has yet to achieve: the so-called universal value that all lives matter.

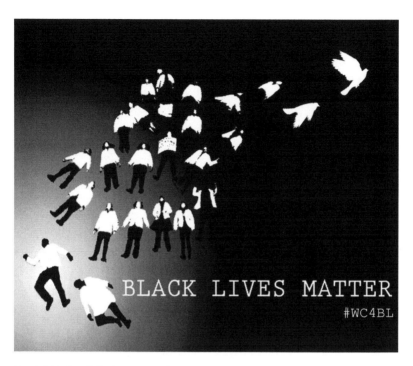

Figure 7. White Coats for Black Lives, *WC4BL flyer. Copyright Yakira Teitel, MD, MPH.*

Provocative protest actions, such as die-ins, confront racism dispersed throughout the spaces of everyday life as a means of revealing and refusing anti-black violence. During a die-in, groups of protesters "play dead" in public spaces, lying down en masse in the middle of intersections, train stations, lobbies, classrooms, public squares, and so forth.[102] The momentary overlay of a symbolic mass grave of bodies vividly portrays the biopolitics of disposability at work through the operations of race in the United States.[103] The die-ins are opportunities to publicly mourn the mounting losses of black lives and to reject the unjust threat to be killed that African Americans confront merely by going about their everyday lives. While die-ins are part of a longer history of civil disobedience and protest efforts, the Black Lives Matter mass actions insistently demand witness to the long-standing and ongoing subjection of African Americans to coercive force and exclusion from public life and health. Performing an iteration of the die-in, parts of the medical community have engaged in Black Lives Matter organizing through medical die-ins or "white coat die-ins." Protesters, usually medical students, lie down motionless, as if dead, on hospital and clinical floors, while wearing white coats—what has become the conventional "uniform" of doctors and a symbol (however problematic) of scientific authority, healing, and responsibility for saving lives. Medical die-ins visually reference and reverse power relations and professional roles within the medical establishment: those who are charged with saving lives paradoxically drop dead.

While medical die-ins could be looked at as supporting more resources for customizing biomedicine, the very performative act of the die-in suggests a move away from the medical environment to a more expansive envisioning of racial justice—echoing the movements we cite earlier and the more general range of efforts advanced through community health centers. This momentary refusal to be instrumental to pervasive medical institutional racism—and the effort to link biomedicine to broader social relations—powerfully draws connections between police brutality against blacks and the protocols and practices of the U.S. health care system that have led to poorer health, shorter life expectancies, and inferior medical care for black Americans.[104] The collective action of suspended medical professional operations—of enacting protest as a professional obligation to public health—opens up the potential to address the role of explicit and implicit forms of discrimination and structural racism in clinical learning environments, medical administrative decision-making, medical education curricula, and daily hospital operations that affect not only blacks but the range of minority and poor individuals in the United States. This form of collective action advocates for future abolitionist practices *that refuse to resecure race as the problem*: that reject the racialized biopolitics of health because it "kills, sickens, and provides inadequate care" and that publicly excavate—and mourn—the ruins of nonfuturity that *are* our institutions.[105] And, while the same doctors or medical students might support race-targeted pharmaceuticals and race-based coordinated care, surely what is needed is something more imaginative and visionary than prescriptive and constraining reinstantiations of racial essentialism as the means through which to cultivate life.[106] What remains, then, is the question of how such a *refusal of what is* might translate *in the present moment* into practical efforts toward an *abolitionist biomedicine*—in relation to both care delivery and drug development—to rework the biopresent and pursue alternative biofutures.

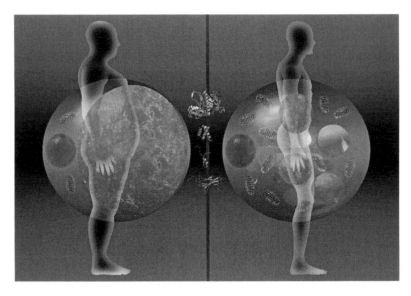

Figure 8. Medical representations of, left, *white fat tissue cell (WAT) and,* right, *brown adipose tissue cell (BAT). Copyright Carol Werner.*

3

Thrive

Fat

*To set the problem in these terms is to imagine a different sense in which
vital phenomena, in their multiplicity and indeterminacy, are political.*

—Monica Greco, "The Politics of Indeterminacy and the Right to Health"

*Obstacles to physical and mental flourishing require other frames for
elaborating contexts of doing, being, and thriving.*

—Lauren Berlant, "Slow Death"

Within the dominant logics and epistemologies of the Western imaginary,
fatness and the vital materiality of fat itself have been viewed negatively.
Fat bodies are "constructed (and discriminated against) as being unhealthy,
ugly, and 'out of place,'" and the substance of fat is defined as that which
must be expelled from the body—precisely because it is seen as surplus
and negative waste.[1] Fatness has become synonymous with deviance in
this cultural context, and bodies that are designated as fat are "fragmented,
medicalized, pathologized, and transformed into abject visions of the hor-
ror of flesh itself."[2]

These views on fat are largely based on biomedical claims about the
health risks of being "overweight" or "obese"—terms and normalizing categories that are themselves open to questioning.[3] However, such views are
also associated with moral and aesthetic judgments that are made concerning what a fat body is said to represent, such as laziness, lack of control,
asexuality, and undesirability. In distinction, what is taken as the ideal or
normative body is a "tight and 'bolted down' form," in other words, "a body
that is protected against eruption and whose internal processes are under
control."[4] Such ideas can inarguably be attributed to post-Enlightenment
binaries that position control/chaos, order/disorder, bounded/unbounded,
and self/body as oppositional categories. Within such a context, fat bodies
are equated with bodily chaos and being out of bounds, and the "fat self"

is seen—based on Cartesian logic—to have lost authority over the body it is meant to master.[5] Beyond being viewed negatively, fat has been associated with the failure to thrive: that is, as that which prevents the body and life itself from flourishing and, ultimately, as that which portends death.[6] Indeed, as Le'a Kent has noted, "the fat body represents the corporeality and inevitable death of all bodies.... The fat body is linked with death, and allowing fat into the body is thought to inevitably court death."[7]

This threat to life is governed in the biomedical and broader social sphere through a diverse range of practices and interventions that comprise biocultures of anti-obesity. This chapter explores how initiatives within biocultures of anti-obesity are ostensibly concerned with life-making and proposes that such efforts (whether practical or rhetorical) are predicated on the *affirmation to thrive*: to flourish, to improve, to be healthy. In the context of obesity, this is a regulatory affirmation that calls for the individual to adopt an entrepreneurial subjectivity: to be strong, to eat well, and to make good choices.[8] What we show, however, is that this supposedly positive affirmation supports a negative social reality—that is *anti/against* fatness—in which those who are deemed as fat or obese are positioned as failed social subjects. Moreover, anti-obesity interventions create or sustain deathly conditions that actually curtail life or threaten vitality itself. Namely, the practices we analyze do little to address the structural conditions marked by racism and economic disadvantage that contribute to escalating levels of obesity in the United States, and they often enable or are complicit in industry/private-sector exploitation that produces fatness or capitalizes on people who are demarcated as fat.

Despite the seeming overdetermination of fat materiality in anti-obesity discourse and interventions, fat has no ontological status. Rather, the way fat signifies—the meaning it accrues and the status it holds—depends on the domain in which it comes to be known and operate. Calling on the quote with which the chapter opens, fat must be understood, then, as a vital phenomenon that is multiple and indeterminate. In exploring the multiplicity of fat materiality and how fat is viewed, we shift away from obesity governance to examine a second case study related to fat: the relatively new deployment of fat/adipose tissue in biocultures of stem cell science.

In this biocultural context, fat has moved from being a category of surplus waste to an object of biovalue. For Catherine Waldby, *biovalue* refers to "the yield of vitality produced by the biotechnical reformulation of living processes,"[9] while Nikolas Rose uses the term to refer to "the value extracted from the vital properties of living processes."[10] Fat is distinct from other forms of excess body material, such as ova, sperm, and embryos, precisely because where it is deemed excessive, it is usually pathologized. It is also distinct, however, from other forms of pathologized bodily waste (such as feces, urine, and pus) because of its potential utility in a therapeutic context.[11] Fat becomes biovalue in the domain of regenerative medicine because its very vitality—its live-ness, malleability, and capacity—can be harnessed and redeployed, and this takes place because the adipose-derived stem cells (ADSCs) found in fat tissue have been identified as biological material that enables life to thrive.

The affirmation to thrive is clearly also at work in this domain. What we see, however, is a perverse reversal. In biocultures of anti-obesity, the affirmation to thrive is predicated on the eradication of fat—through entrepreneurial subjectivity. In biocultures of stem cell therapy, however, the *affirmation to thrive works to affirm life through the animation of fat and the growth it enables.* An epistemological shift occurs wherein fat is valued as a potential form of entrepreneurial materiality that can facilitate life-making. But, though the thriving enabled by fat—through stem cell proliferation— represents a new horizon in the biomedical fostering of life, we show that it also solidifies inequitable distributions of life based on economic access; it converts the body into a speculative asset; and it can threaten life itself. Ultimately, what becomes evident is that fat—and specifically the fat cell—is differently valued according to the body in which it is located and the biocultural arena in which it circulates. Furthermore, fat at once represents the impediment to *and* means through which to thrive, and in both domains or biocultural arenas, fat kills, or is said to kill—but offers the material ground for exploitation. In concluding the chapter, we ask, how might we work against the death effects of the affirmation to thrive and pursue more inclusive and socially accountable ways to thrive?

Biocultures of Anti-obesity and the Abject Matter of Fat

The World Health Organization has declared obesity a global epidemic. In a recent fact sheet, the organization claimed that in 2016, more than 1.9 billion adults aged eighteen years and older were overweight. Of these, more than 650 million were obese. Thirty-nine percent of adults aged eighteen years and older were overweight in 2016, and 13 percent were obese.[12] The Centers for Disease Control and Prevention (CDC) has estimated that 39.8

percent of adults and 18.5 percent of children are currently obese in the United States.[13] Both organizations claim that the worldwide prevalence of obesity more than doubled between 1980 and 2014. Adding further complexity to U.S. figures, data from the National Health and Nutrition Examination Survey 2009–10 stated that more than two in three adults are considered to be overweight or obese; more than one in three adults are considered to be obese; more than one in twenty adults are considered to have extreme obesity; about one-third of children and adolescents ages six to nineteen are considered to be overweight or obese; and more than one in six children and adolescents ages six to nineteen are considered to be obese.[14]

Fat alarmism is presumably due, in no small part, to the fact that fat has been provisionally associated with a raft of medical conditions, such as type 2 diabetes, heart disease, high blood pressure, nonalcoholic fatty liver disease, osteoarthritis, multiple types of cancer (including breast, colon, endometrial, and kidney cancers), and stroke.[15] As early as 2001, this alarmism led then U.S. Surgeons General C. Everett Koop and David Satcher to declare a national "war against obesity," to avert what they announced as the three hundred thousand "excess deaths" related to fat.[16] To launch the war, they and the Health and Human Services Secretary held a press conference and, to motivate everyone watching, stated that "all Americans—as their patriotic duty—should lose 10 pounds."[17] In 2006, Surgeon General Richard Carmona vilified persons classified as "obese" as "domestic bioterrorists," thereby situating the "obese" individual as a legitimate "enemy target" in the "war"—a war that resonated within a larger nationalist, patriotic narrative post-9/11.[18] And, in an act that cemented the mounting panic over fatness, the American Medical Association passed Resolution 420 in 2013, which was short and to the point: "that our American Medical Association recognize obesity as a *disease state* with multiple pathophysiological aspects *requiring a range of interventions* to advance obesity treatment and prevention."[19] This new label—"disease state"—is predicted to affect the way obesity is identified and treated and was deemed an appropriate classification because of the heightened prevalence of obesity, its threat to health, and increases in obesity-related health care expenditure, which is said to average $200 billion annually in the United States.[20]

These various forms of moral and medical panic over obesity have been reflected in what the American Medical Association called for: a proliferation of interventions and processes that aim to manage the problem of obesity and promote weight-related well-being—to administer fatness.

Such interventions ostensibly labor to optimize the life of individuals and populations in and against the threat of fat. Collectively, they can be said to endeavor to make the population live more, and thereby they act as instantiations of the affirmation to thrive. In the first instance, all individuals are encouraged to thrive through regulating themselves in relation to what is viewed as excess weight—to affirm their own life through monitoring and minimizing the risks associated with fat. We see such incitements daily—and hear them in thunderous symphony[21]—on our televisions, in food advertising, in public service announcements related to health, and in our doctor's offices. As Pirkko Markula has noted, individual citizens are now asked to take on primary responsibility for health in the face of fatness: "to locate themselves within the BMI [Body Mass Index] scale, to confess to being fat and to seek the appropriate bodily discipline (diet and exercise) to avoid becoming an economic burden for society."[22] Put another way, the American ideal of what Kathryn Pauly Morgan has called "carnal governmentality" is "a vigilant community of disciplined (and self-disciplining), compliant individuals—totalized by being sorted mathematically [and] . . . weighed and measured into discrete categories of normalcy and hierarchies of obesity-pathology."[23]

Should individually led forms of prevention fail, one key way of intervening against obesity is via the biomedical approach, which focuses on biological factors of obesity. More generally, in the biomedical realm, genetic and early life factors are examined in relation to obesity, as are prenatal nutrition, biofood activities, and the role of fat tissue itself. Epidemiology, a branch of biomedical science, concentrates on regional prevalence of obesity, secular trends, risk factors, burden of illness related to obesity, and possible determinants. Importantly, the biomedical approach defines obesity via the BMI scale (a measurement system that has been widely criticized) and views "abnormal feeding behavior" as the primary cause of obesity.[24] For instance, the National Institutes of Health states,

> Overweight and obesity result from an energy imbalance. The body needs a certain amount of energy (calories) from food to keep up basic life functions. Body weight tends to remain the same when the number of calories eaten equals the number of calories the body uses or "burns." Over time, *when people eat and drink more calories than they burn, the energy balance tips toward weight gain, overweight, and obesity.*[25]

In response, biomedical approaches concentrate on nonsurgical and surgical treatment methods to reduce weight. These methods include the use of anti-obesity pharmaceutical agents ("diet pills" like orlistat and sibutramine), the monitoring of diet, and—as an intervention of last resort—obesity surgery (gastric banding, bypass, and sleeve surgeries). Such biomedical protocols both biopolitically administer the population and discipline individual bodies: they are offered both as ways to regularize the mass of bodies that comprise the population and as techniques to "correct" and normalize the singular body.

A second key way of intervening into and administering obesity is through the public health approach, which generally draws on biomedical framings and understandings of fatness. This approach provides a population-based account of obesity (calling on epidemiological evidence) and pursues public policy changes that are important in the attempt to reduce the toll of poor diet, physical inactivity, and extreme weight: such efforts are clearly biopolitical in that they represent the calculated management of life of the masses that comprise the population.[26] The public health approach concentrates primarily on prevention via public education around making positive food choices, exercise protocols, and general lifestyle choices. But public health authorities have also taken a more hands-on governing approach, stressing the need for food labeling, and in certain jurisdictions (such as New York City), they have succeeded in placing taxes on foods that are deemed to contribute to the rise of obesity. Intersecting with public health initiatives are state interventions against both childhood and adult obesity, which constitute a third form of obesity administration. For instance, in 2008, the Georgia State Senate passed a bill mandating that schoolchildren be weighed twice a year by school officials, New York City sends home "fitnessgrams," and Philadelphia delivers "obesity report cards" to the parents of schoolchildren (six states in total have laws that require individualized assessment of children). In extreme cases, the state has forcibly removed children from their parents' custody, using fatness alone as evidence of parental neglect (two reputable cases would be the Alexander Draper and Anamarie Regino cases).[27] A final key way obesity is administered is via the diet and fitness industry that supports weight reduction. This industry is composed of proprietary weight reduction diets, diet facilities, food companies, pharmaceutical companies, diet and fitness book and magazine companies, personal trainers and health clubs, exercise programs, personal chefs, and so on. Estimates calculate the annual revenue of the U.S. weight loss industry at $72 billion per year (as of 2018), highlighting both the reach of weight administration and its financialization.[28]

While many of these interventions may attempt to move toward mitigating unhealthiness and death, they simultaneously advance *and compromise* the ability to thrive in a general sense and to reduce obesity more specifically. Such compromise can be seen in the very *individualization of obesity*—where fat and fatness are situated in biocultures of anti-obesity as only-ever-abject and as the materialization of individual failure. There are two important points to be made here, then: corpulence can never be imagined or circulate in the social sphere in a benign sense, and the healthy body—now only interpellated as slim—has come to signify the morally worthy citizen. It is due to these two notions that, as Lauren Berlant has argued, "the epidemic concept is not a neutral description, but always a contribution to ongoing mechanisms of social distinction. Who's degenerate, who's competent, and who's out of and in control."[29] And it is precisely because both the supposed origin and answer to this epidemic is the atomized subject that obesity is individualized.

This individualization of obesity (and fatness more generally) is clearly evident in biomedical approaches, where the individual's eating practices and body become governable and targets of intervention. The body, here, is divorced from its social context and subject to a form of power that, as Michel Foucault claims, is "centered on the body as a machine: its disciplining, the optimization of its capabilities, the extortion of its forces, the parallel increase of its usefulness and its docility, its integration into systems of efficient and economic controls."[30] Thus, while biomedicine operates at the level of population in the case of obesity (to regularize the social body en masse through inaugurating and disseminating practices of normalizing governmentality, such as the BMI), it more tangibly operates at the level of individual subjects to discipline the body and its size. Yet, biomedical approaches—which generally operate as adjuncts to lifestyle interventions (exercise, changing eating habits, etc.)—curtail vitality in myriad ways and threaten the ability to thrive in the same moment that they supposedly offer the means by which to eradicate fat. For instance, the weight loss pharmaceutical orlistat (Xenical), sold also in a low-dose form over the counter in the United States (as Alli), was marketed in the early 2000s under the slogan "Lose Weight. Gain Life." But the drug compromises daily life through its most common side effects, which include oily rectal discharge; passing gas with oily discharge; urgent need to have a bowel movement; oily or fatty stools; increased number of bowel movements; being unable to control bowel movements.[31] The drug also dissolves other fat-soluble substances in the body, including vitamins A, D, E, K, and beta-carotene, depleting the body over time; it has the potential long-term effects of producing kidney and liver damage; and it has been found to produce (in rats) high numbers of aberrant crypt foci colon lesions, which are believed to be one of the earliest precursors of colon cancer.[32] Similarly, the weight loss drug sibutramine (Reductil) has the following side effects: dry mouth, nausea, strange taste in the mouth, upset stomach, constipation, trouble sleeping, dizziness, drowsiness, menstrual cramps/pain, headache, flushing, and joint or muscle pain. It also paradoxically increases appetite and was withdrawn from the market in 2010 in a number of countries (including the United States) because of findings that it significantly increased cardiovascular disorders, resulting in excess deaths.

Surgical biomedical approaches to obesity are no less troubling. What are collectively known as bariatric surgeries (including gastric bypass, adjustable gastric banding, and sleeve gastrectomy) commonly result in what is known as dumping syndrome, a condition stemming from corporeal changes after these surgeries and marked by "dizziness, palpitations, lightheadedness, nausea, and the sudden urge to vomit or defecate in response to foods with high carbohydrate content or sugar."[33] And, while weight loss is reported in most cases, acute complications associated with bariatric surgeries (which occur in 5 to 10 percent of patients, depending on the procedure, patient risk, age, and condition) include hemorrhage, obstruction, anastomotic leaks, infection, arrhythmias, pulmonary emboli, and rhabdomyolysis. Longer-term complications included neuropathies due to nutritional deficiencies, internal hernias, anastomotic stenoses, and emotional disorders.[34] Despite these complications and death effects, bariatric surgeries are generally characterized in terms of "biomedical success," and while this success might be attributed to surgical skill, it still unilaterally requires individual postoperative compliance and ongoing discipline, which situates any failure to lose weight or the regaining of fat—the failure to thrive—as internal to the individual.

Individualization is also at work in public health approaches to obesity. For instance, in a fact sheet on obesity subtitled "What Can Be Done," the CDC instructs people to do the following: "eat more fruits and vegetables and fewer foods high in fat and sugar; drink more water instead of sugary drinks; watch less television; support breastfeeding; promote policies and programs at school, work, and in the community to make the healthy choice the easy choice; be more physically active."[35] Lastly, we see the individualization of obesity and efforts to intervene against fatness in governmental efforts to address fatness. Punitive governmental measures to disincentivize weight gain were put in place, for example, in the U.S. health care reform law of 2010 (the Affordable Care Act, ACA), which allows employers to charge obese workers 30 to 50 percent more for health insurance if they decline to participate in a qualified wellness program. The ACA also persuades Medicare and Medicaid enrollees to see a primary care physician about losing weight and funds community demonstration programs for weight loss.[36] In such programs, employees who fail particular health biometrics (such as meeting a specific BMI target) incur a penalty or, if they meet the standard, receive a benefit. In another example, the Federal Action Plan of May 2010, released by the White House Task Force on Childhood Obesity (following a memorandum issued by former U.S. President Obama), also largely directed the incitement to eradicate fat—to reduce the tide of escalating obesity rates—at the individual level.[37] The plan, which was in part actualized as the Let's Move! campaign spearheaded by Michelle Obama, laid out five key pillars or action areas. Two of these pillars again stressed personal responsibility in relation to minimizing childhood obesity specifically. The first, "Early Childhood," mentions the need to reduce chemical "obesogens" (the term given to a host of chemicals that may promote weight gain and obesity), but only in the context of individual activity (such as microwaving plastic baby bottles) and only after noting two behavioral elements—self-regulation regarding preconception weight and prenatal care and self-disciplining in terms of breast-feeding. The second, "Empowering Parents and Caregivers," stresses that the fundamental responsibility of child health and development rests with the parents (stating "children learn from the *choices* adults make"). Such language effectively deflects attention away from the limited capacities certain people have to "choose," which in turn shape consumption, eating, and broader behaviors.[38]

These various ways of individualizing obesity are problematic because, as we have outlined, they potentially subject people to numerous deathly conditions and forms of punitive administration. More than this, however, the very individualization of fatness ultimately compromises life because it does little to address the impersonal etiologies and structural conditions—broader sociopolitical, geographic, and economic factors— that have led to increasing rates of obesity that affect both individuals and entire communities.

First, what is overshadowed through the relentless forms of individualization outlined here are the ways that fatness and obesity are products of the political economy of food in the United States (and, of course, in numerous other countries throughout the world). As many critical food and fat studies scholars, along with antipoverty and antihunger activists, have insisted, people live in a toxic environment in the United States, where too much food is produced.[39] Indeed, there is an infinite supply of what are known as "durable foods" (for example, corn, soy, sugar, wheat) because of the generous support of state agricultural subsidies, and it is these commodities that are then used to produce highly processed, high-caloric "junk." Served in supersized portions to overworked, time-poor neoliberal subjects—who are confronted daily with a plethora of cheap, easy-to-access, nutrient-deficient food—this junk food is all around us and is "feeding" the nation. In the context of this obesogenic environment, making "good choices" is impossible for many. Moreover, alongside infinite supply, food marketing induces people to eat more, and as Julie Guthman and Melanie DuPuis have noted, in our contemporary context, we are encouraged to consume greater and greater quantities to be ideal neoliberal citizens: "eating becomes the embodiment of that which today's society holds sacred: consumption. We buy and eat to be good subjects."[40]

Second, focusing on fatness and obesity as individual and individualized phenomena obscures the ways they are conditioned by—and often the product of—material deprivation based on race and class (and their intersections). In other words, fatness and obesity can be a predicament of poverty, and as such, they can eventuate as the corporeal *effects* or the *materialization* of deprivation. Black Americans and Latinx most particularly bear this bodily burden, highlighting the racialization of fatness in the United States. According to recent figures from the National Institutes of Health, overweight and obesity affect 78.8 percent of Latinx and 76.7 percent of blacks, compared to 66.7 percent of whites. Almost 50 percent of blacks and more than one in three Latinx (39.1 percent) are considered to be obese (as opposed to 34.3 percent of their white counterparts), and extreme obesity affects more than one in ten blacks (13.1 percent), compared to 5.7 percent of whites and 5 percent of Latinx.[41]

The racial disparities in these figures are the result of complex histories of disenfranchisement, segregation, lack of access to resources, and inadequate allocation of resources related to achieving food security and health optimization more generally. For instance, many lower-income minorities experience impediments to spatial access to food, which manifests in extreme forms as food deserts.[42] As the Racial Justice Project has noted, low-income minority communities are less likely to have access to super-markets than nonminority communities, and what they do have access to—smaller grocery stores—carry less varied and higher-priced items than those found in other communities. In Washington, D.C., for example, "the District's two lowest income neighborhoods, which are overwhelmingly African-American, have one supermarket for every 70,000 residents compared to 1 supermarket for approximately every 12,000 residents in two of the District's highest income and predominantly white neighborhoods."[43] Given that limited access to nutritionally rich food potentially impacts rates of obesity (making people hungry, fat, and undernourished[44]), what we see here again is the way race and racism might "cut" the biopolitical fostering of life. At the same time, recent research in epigenetics—which focuses on the ways environments affect gene expression—has established that obesity might have other racialized etiologies not accounted for by behavioral or food access approaches. Exposure to certain agricultural chemicals (that act as endocrine disruptors), chronic stress and accompanying cortisol circulation (which has been shown to result from experiencing institutional racism), and generationally passed-on malnutrition have all been associated with escalated rates of obesity in minority populations. Epigenetic processes can be heritable across several generations and highlight another form of "letting die."[45] In the context of these factors, we see clearly that minorities have been and continue to be unequally incorporated into biological citizenship, resulting in what Didier Fassin has called "bioinequality" or what Matthew Sparke has theorized as "biological subcitizenship."[46] In such a context, focusing on individual "good choices" only further compounds racialized disparities through stigmatization—if they fail to do so—and overwhelms the reality that, as Berlant has eloquently stated, "morbidity, the embodiment toward death as a way of life, marks out slow death as what there is" for many people of color in the United States.[47]

In addition to acknowledging how the political economy of food and material deprivation contribute to fatness and obesity, we must be aware of (and contest) the ways that many interventions against the threat of fat can sustain or indeed be complicit in private-sector or industry exploitation of fatness—producing fatness, capitalizing on those demarcated as fat, and/or exacerbating death. Put another way, there is money to be made in making people fat, and fat bodies have become rich sites of financial extraction or points of accumulation within neocapitalist frameworks. Private industry is implicated here in numerous ways. We have already discussed how the food industry is complicit in fattening the nation and sustaining obesity. So, in the most obvious sense, this industry makes money out of creating products that make people fat, but it also then sells products to people that help slim them down—in the form of diet or calorie-restricted foods and beverages. The biggest market here is not the morbidly obese but all those individuals who have been made conscious of their weight through the relentless normalizing technologies and knowledges associated with fatness that pervade biocultures of anti-obesity. The pharmaceutical industry—which funds a great portion of obesity research—sets and lowers "at risk" levels of glucose, cholesterol, and other obesity-related biomarkers, enabling drug manufacturers to sell more medications to more people and exponentially increase profits. The life sciences are making genetics, microbiota, and stem cells, as they relate to obesity, sites of investment.[48] Media profits from obesity through creating entertainment: *The Biggest Loser, Celebrity Fit Club, Thintervention, Extreme Weight Loss,* and *Fit to Fat to Fit.* The diet industry pumps out new proprietary weight loss regimes and fitness programs at an ever-increasing rate. And, finally, the new bodily forms created through weight loss surgeries have "created a new market for everything from new forms of plastic surgeries to remove post-weight-loss 'redundant' skin, nutritional supplements and specialty foods, to beaded medic-alert bracelets and weight-loss surgery scrapbooks."[49]

What becomes evident, ultimately, is that the affirmation to thrive in relation to obesity is fraught. The ability to thrive—at both the individual and communal levels—is limited and the lives of many are curtailed, thereby exposing the "death function in the economy of biopower."[50] In neoliberal times, this is only exacerbated by a financial imperative that affirms an altogether different operation: the ability of industry and private-sector businesses to thrive economically—to thrive off fat and forms of premature death.

Biocultures of Stem Cell Therapy: Where Fat Is "Liquid Gold"

The way fat is understood and administered in biocultures of anti-obesity relies on the notion that fat is negative waste that kills and that such fat needs to be eradicated. Yet, paradoxically, in both biomedicine and broader social arenas, fat has undergone a reversal of status. Fat has come to signify something altogether else: it is a substance that can be harvested, harnessed, and redeployed therapeutically to facilitate corporeal repair or the extension—indeed, the proliferation—of life itself. Rather than being a threat, then, fat is viewed as the possible new horizon of life. This epistemological reversal is not, however, a simple inversion of status. Rather, as Catherine Waldby and Robert Mitchell have argued, it is only because a tissue is designated as waste—a part of the body to be expelled—that it can be put to another use.[51] In the case of fat, it is only because it is classified as surplus and as a substance that can be wasted that it can be reevaluated and redeployed in another context. Put another way, value is facilitated by the tissue being categorized as waste. It is, then, a perverse reversal, in that fat has to be waste (and wasted) to be valued. Moreover, in biocultures of stem cell science, this value can only be secured once fat has been removed from the body. That is, fat can only be converted into value in abstracted form, and once it is liberated from the body, it can circulate as a form of *entrepreneurial material* that can be used to make individuals live (more). What we see, then, is that the materiality of fat—as a phenomenon—is multiple and indeterminate, and in certain biomedical contexts, it is called into the service of the affirmation to thrive, as the means through which to thrive, and individuals are encouraged to think of their own fat as that which can affirm life.

The therapeutic use of fat is by no means a new invention. For example, for more than a century, surgeons have used patients' own fat, along with muscle and skin, to enlarge and reshape breasts following mastectomy. German physician Vincent Czerny performed the first documented case using such methods in 1895, when he transplanted a lipoma (a benign tumor comprising fat tissue) from the lumbar region to reconstruct a breast.[52] Since then, in what might be referred to as first-generation deployments of adipose tissue, fat has been redistributed to other parts of the body for therapeutic repair. We see this in forms of fat transfer and fat grafting, where preexisting fat is moved from one part of the body to another. Yet, such uses of fat have been limited in that they can only achieve a point-to-point substitution.

The relatively recent discovery of stem cells in fat tissue has, however, altered the limitation previously associated with fat and has been a eureka moment in biotechnological developments.[53] Indeed, new possibilities for life have been found "hidden in a pair of love handles."[54] As UCLA pediatric plastic surgeon Marc Hedrick has noted, "fat is not the tissue we once thought. For too long it was seen as something to be removed and tossed away [following most forms of lipoaspiration]. . . . We weren't seeing its potential. We now know that it's not just spare tissue."[55] What is so promising about this discovery is that fat-derived stem cells—what are known as adipose-derived stem cells (ADSCs)—can be used within tissue engineering and regenerative medicine to *regenerate* injured parts of the body and thus enable corporeal renewal. As such, with the identification of stem cells in fat, the surplus or residual becomes regenerative and emergent, thereby expanding the material and biotechnological possibilities and capacities of fat and exponentially increasing its *value.*

ADSCs are adult stem cells. Both embryonic stem cells and adult stem cells renew themselves in a process of self-renewal or morphogenesis. However, while embryonic stem cells are pluripotent, meaning that they are "blank" or undifferentiated cells that hold the potential to give rise to any type of cell, adult stem cells have a specific physiological function—to replenish the cells in their home tissues as needed. Adult stem cells are multipotent: these cells can give rise to different kinds of cells in their home tissues through entering normal differentiation pathways, but they do not normally generate cell types outside of their particular tissues or cell lineages. Despite this restricted developmental potential, adult stem cells can be manipulated in vitro to differentiate into different types of cells, including cells of different germ origin; and in vivo, the same changes can be seen when these stem cells are transplanted into a tissue environment other than their tissue of origin.

Adult stem cells have been identified in many organs and tissues, including brain matter, bone marrow, peripheral blood, blood vessels, skeletal muscle, skin, teeth, heart, gut, liver, ovarian epithelium, and testis.[56] And, while the stem cells found in bone marrow have been considered the gold standard of adult stem cells, they are difficult to source, and such sourcing is achieved only through complicated and painful procedures. Finding stem cells in fat has, then, altered the terrain of stem cell science, and ADSC technologies/therapeutics are increasingly becoming the focus of clinical trials in regenerative medicine (with the U.S. government registering in excess of 300 national and international clinical trials involving ADSCs in application for a wide variety of pathologies).[57] The reasons for this heightened interest are threefold: harvesting stem cells from fat circumvents the ethical minefield associated with using stem cells from embryos—because fat, unlike the embryo, is seen as inconsequential tissue; it is easy to source—liposuction is a relatively common and uncomplicated procedure, and more than four hundred thousand liposuctions are conducted per year in the United States alone, with each yielding between one hundred milliliters and more than three liters of fat;[58] and, beyond being expendable, nearly everyone has some fat that they can spare. Moreover, fat has been identified as the richest source of adult stem cells, and these cells have been found not only to generate adipose tissue but also to differentiate successfully—through inducing processes—into bone, cartilage, muscle, skin, and nerves.[59]

To date, adipose-derived stem cells have specifically been imagined as "breast-making gold," and breast reconstruction using ADSC therapy was the first major form of applied fat stem cell therapy in humans.[60] That ADSC therapeutics developed in the context of breast reconstruction may be due to the fact that breasts are seen as inconsequential to the laboring body; that is, breasts are not required to "work" for the individual's body to survive.[61] It is considerably easier and more strategic, then, to clear regulatory hurdles through conducting stem cell research in relation to breasts rather than other tissue or organs. But despite the fact that breasts are seen as relatively inconsequential within the general taxonomy of corporeal significance, ADSC therapy represents an important way through which individuals might reimagine and materialize the body after breast cancer surgery—by deploying fat to produce an *emergent* breasted materiality, that is, a breast that arises or emerges from the genesis of cells and the interaction of these cells within the biological organism of the human body.

Two companies have been significant in the development of ADSC therapy in relation to breast reconstruction. The first is the San Diego–based biotech company Cytori Therapeutics, which has developed what it calls the RESTORE procedure.[62] This procedure involves harvesting fat through liposuction and injecting this fat into what Cytori calls the Celution system—a patented machine that processes the tissue, extracts the patient's regenerative cells, and concentrates them into a pellet. These concentrated stem cells are then combined with some of the liposuctioned fat cells to create a liquid suspension, which is then deposited back into the breast site, creating a biological mesh that is subsequently incorporated into preexisting tissue. The RESTORE procedure is heralded as being more successful than traditional fat grafts because the ADSC-rich suspension increases the growth factor signaling at the interface between the newly grafted tissue and the adjacent vascularized tissue, improving overall incorporation.[63] A second company pursuing ADSC therapy for breast reconstruction is Neopec Pty Ltd., which is Australian-based and funded by the Victorian State Government. Neopec—whose guiding motto is "natural. individual.

forever."—aims to "entice a woman's own regenerative capacity to grow living fat as a substitute for breast reconstruction."[64] The technique developed by the company involves implanting a biodegradable synthetic chamber into the mastectomy site, redirecting blood vessels from under the armpit into the chamber, and injecting the chamber with stem cell–rich lipoaspirate, which will grow to fill the space of the chamber over a period of four to six months.[65] Both of these technologies endeavor to reimagine materiality and enable a supposed return to normative embodiment through the genesis and animation of form itself.

ADSC technologies are indeed promising: they envision (and actualize) the emergence of life through the very thriving of the stem cells found in fat. Registered clinical trials using ADSCs are in the process of exploring how they might enable soft tissue regeneration, musculoskeletal regeneration, cardiovascular regeneration, and nervous system regeneration. Studies have shown that fat stem cells are effective in treating Crohn's disease, pulmonary disease, Parkinson's, and various autoimmune diseases. And, given this potential, Medical and Scientific Advisory Board member Rand McClain sums up the overriding response to this promise of fat: "it really is amazing. The process of extracting stem cells from fat and reintroducing them into the body allows the body the ability, in essence, to heal itself naturally."[66]

Despite this promise, however, ADSC technologies simultaneously present a number of contingencies that are obscured in much of the hype. First, and perhaps most importantly, at the same time that ADSCs are being reimagined as that which can foster life, they also threaten. New technologies using stem cells rely on processes of transformation and growth of tissue through regenerating the transformable—the emergent stem cell. Yet, it is precisely this reliance on cellular thriving and transformation that makes the technology risky: cells might grow or proliferate *too* well, and where the first signs of life can also mark the first sign of death, the excessive vitality of cells might result in the material emergence of cancer.[67] In this vein, studies have demonstrated that ADSCs home in on tumor sites when injected intravenously and that ADSCs are tumor promoting. Furthermore, ADSCs have been shown to promote the invasion and metastasis of breast cancer specifically.[68] These findings suggest that there should be pause before celebrating fat as the fount of life.

Second, such technologies convert the body and the fat it stores into speculative assets. We see this in the sense that ADSC technologies enable individuals to optimize the body and give what Waldby and Mitchell refer to as a "gift of self to self"—by investing a part of their body in their own future and relying on their own corporeal resources for that future.[69] This reliance on the self is part of a broader operation that Rose names "the ethic of active citizenship that has taken place in advanced liberal democracies."[70] Within this ethic, "the maximization of lifestyle, potential, health, and quality of life has become almost obligatory . . . [and individuals are encouraged to] adopt an active, informed, positive, and prudent relation to the future."[71]

That fat has offered this opportunity—new forms of self-reliance and the maximization of life—is particularly evident in the emergence and proliferation of "fat banks," where individuals can store harvested surplus fat through cryopreservation. The premise of this banking is that stored fat can be reanimated at a later point for a range of therapeutic applications—such as repeated breast reconstruction revisions—or it can be kept (supposedly indefinitely) until ADSC research is developed into future clinical practices. Fat banking is, then, a future-oriented storing of promise, as seen in the language deployed by the banks themselves. For example, American CryoStem refers to the fat banking service it provides as "bioinsurance"; BioLife Cell Bank calls on the individual to "Preserve your cells. Preserve yourself"; and a fat bank called Liquid Gold markets its facility through the slogan "invest/save/withdraw." Advanced Cosmetic Surgery of New York makes a more ambitious and forceful claim: "Storing your Adult Stem Cells has the potential of one day SAVING YOUR LIFE!" (it is only in the disclaimer at the bottom of the page that we are informed that "medical treatments using adult stem cells are still under development").[72]

With fat banking, the promise and value of fat are spectacularly financialized, showing that subjects are being called on to "pay good money to buy back . . . [their] own bodily waste after it [has] . . . been processed through the infrastructure of commodity capitalism."[73] BioLife Cell Bank, as a case in point, previously offered two major banking packages—a "fat (adipose) banking package" and a "stem cell banking package"—with pricing for processing and storing starting at around $2,000 per year.[74] Corporations are thus also employing adipose tissue as a speculative asset and converting the (always potentially) latent corporeal capital of fat into economic capital, a fact that is perhaps most clearly evidenced by the explosion of stem cell clinics worldwide and the burgeoning of stem cell tourism. The National Stem Cell Foundation of Australia refers to such practices as a form of "cowboy culture," in that biotech companies and biomedical practitioners are reaping huge financial profits from therapies that are currently often unregulated and unproven.[75] Promising to cure a range of pathologies—from stroke, muscular dystrophy, and spinal cord injury to Alzheimer's—these clinics (which are featured on stem cell tourism routes in, for instance, locales like Kazakhstan, China, Mexico, and Argentina) prey on people desperate for a cure and willing to pay up to $400,000 for a chance of recovery.[76] Fundamentally, however, fat and the body are positioned in ADSC technologies as speculative assets *of and for* the individual. This framing, in turn, individualizes disease—as the property of particular bodies—and positions the solution to disease as also residing in the individual's body. The risk in such a framing is that attention will be redirected away from looking at broader social etiologies of disease and finding clinical solutions that would benefit (and be accessible by) wider publics.

Third, and related to the preceding point, ADSC technologies encourage and enable the conversion of the liberal subject into the entrepreneurial neoliberal market actor—one who can direct their own restoration, through fat. Problematically, this means that fat gets to be valued and remediated only by those *already privileged* within circuits of capital and broader relations of power. To take breast reconstruction using fat as a case in point (given that it is currently one of the main applications for fat technologies), the teleological end goal of realizing the (always vexed) promise of corporeal repair is conditioned from the outset by racial disparities in breast cancer incidence rates, diagnosis, and survival. According to the U.S. National Center for Health Statistics, death rates from breast cancer among African American women were 39 percent higher than they were among white women in 2015—representing the lowest five-year survival across all racial groups.[77] This trend continues and can be largely attributed to lower frequency of mammograms and early screening, lack of insurance and/ or access to health care, and the "unequal receipt of prompt, high-quality treatment."[78] If health is unable to be divorced from patterns of structural racism and social and economic disenfranchisement, and minority women are dying at increased rates, then corporeal repair is always already a foreclosed dream for some. This dream is further delimited by the fact that even if women survive the disease, there are discrepancies in terms of options to access breast reconstruction technologies—and specifically those using fat. Significant predictors of immediate reconstruction are white race and private insurance. Significant predictors of no reconstruction are diabetes, obesity, black race, and Medicaid.[79] Cost is also clearly prohibitive: the average cost of reconstruction surgery involving autologous fat transfer procedures runs $50,000 to $100,000 (without insurance), and, while ADSC technologies for breast reconstruction are not yet commercially available, it is anticipated that their price tag will be at least that of—if not more than—traditional methods. As such, the potential to pursue repair or restoration—to thrive through fat—needs to be understood as a privilege enjoyed by a largely white, upper-middle-class, insured population.[80]

Other Frames of Being, Doing, and Thriving

Biocultures of anti-obesity and biocultures of stem cell science are diametrically opposed in their approach to fat and in how they epistemologically order and value fat. In the first biocultural arena, fat is said to kill. In the second, it is said to offer the possibility of corporeal renewal and life extension through fat stem cell proliferation. The affirmation to thrive is predicated in the first arena on the idea that individuals must eradicate fat through entrepreneurial activity, yet in the second, the affirmation to thrive is based on harnessing and redirecting the cellular potential of fat as entrepreneurial material—to reproduce life, whether that be of the cell itself or of the patient/body more generally. In both contexts, however, thriving is contoured by ideologies and discourses of self-reliance, individual responsibility (in light of declining state support and increasing privatization), and self-enhancement/optimization. As we have explored in numerous ways throughout the preceding chapters, these logics condition contemporary approaches to health: health has become increasingly individualized and that which individuals must be responsible for; individuals are encouraged to maximize their lives through established and emerging biomedical and broader health protocols; and, connected to this, individuals are increasingly encouraged to consume health-related (or purportedly health-enhancing) goods and services to be ideal citizens—to exercise "choice" as a form of freedom, while at the same time expanding markets.[81]

Additionally, in both biocultural arenas, the affirmation to thrive can curtail life and be deadly. In biocultures of anti-obesity, biomedicalized governance of fatness can and does endanger the health and well-being of individuals demarcated as "fat"—whether that be through the effects of biomedical interventions themselves or through forms of punitive administration. The individualization of obesity—and the entrepreneurial subjectivity advanced in anti-obesity initiatives—obscures broader sociopolitical, environmental, geographical, and economic etiologies of fatness and facilitates their continuation. Additionally, the lucrative market in fat production/ fatness facilitates the "letting die" of many. In biocultures of stem cell science, calls to exploit the entrepreneurial materiality of fat individualize the body as a speculative asset, deepen and secure inequitable distributions of life chances, and potentially invite the material threat of cancer. Within the context of such let-die operations, the question remains, how might we work against these logics and practices and pursue other ways to thrive?

In the first instance, it will be necessary to question and work against the largely economic premise of what underscores the discourse of the "obesity epidemic" and its accompanying governing strategies: those financial logics that both propel escalating levels of obesity, on one hand, and benefit from those levels, on the other. In the second instance, finding other ways to thrive will also, as Kathleen LeBesco has noted, require looking "more closely at paths to wellbeing that abstain from the kind of carrot and stick model that beats down those it preemptively deems unhealthy."[82] One such possible path is the Health at Every Size (HAES) movement, which works against the pathologizing biomedical model of obesity. The movement advances principles like promoting bodily diversity, valuing pleasurable and individually appropriate forms of physical activity that are not aimed solely at weight loss, and "eating in a flexible and attuned manner that values pleasure and honors internal cues of hunger, satiety, and appetite, while respecting the social conditions that frame eating options."[83] In supporting such commitments, HAES seeks to broaden typical definitions of health— in relation to weight—beyond the restrictive terrain on which it now rests. One such example is the HAES-affiliated I STAND photo campaign. Developed by Marilyn Wann, individuals take photographs of themselves standing up to negative fat discourse to challenge and change anti-fat social prejudice—particularly against children.[84]

Another possible path is to view eating as what Berlant has called "self-medication," while at the same time reworking what self-medication means.[85] To self-medicate in relation to food is not, in this understanding, directed toward "health at any cost" or health as the end point or teleological goal of human subjectivity—where it is viewed as an individual attribute, as located in the body, and as fixed and measurable in relation to a norm. Rather, self-medicating through food might be a way to make things better, to define health in terms of affirming comfort, belonging, conviviality, and enjoyment. Understood in this way, self-medicating is not a negative. Rather, as Berlant notes, "it extends being in the world enjoyably and,

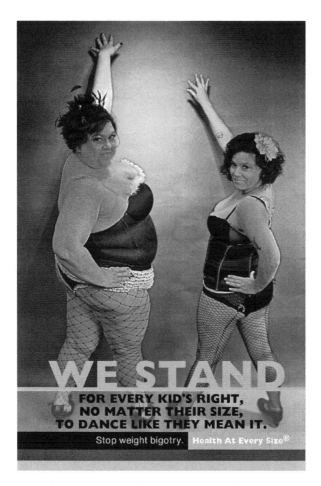

Figure 9. *Kentucky Fried Woman and Starr69. Photograph by Jen Gilomen. Courtesy of I STAND campaign creator Marilyn Wann.*

usually, undramatically."[86] A tangible example here would be to think about health through culinary care as an alternative way to thrive. Emily Yates-Doerr and Megan A. Carney have examined how Latin American kitchens are such sites of culinary care—sharing stories of how women redefine food and feeding as pleasure, where pleasure is "both a means to and expression of health."[87] Their study outlines how women care for and through food: preparing food might be a way to nourish social ties, a way to build strong relationships, a means through which to support local growers and know

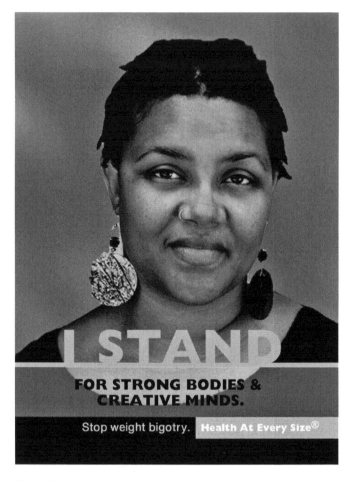

Figure 10. Erin Upchurch. Photograph by Taira Crockett. Courtesy of I STAND campaign creator Marilyn Wann.

the conditions under which food is grown. Individual needs and individualized notions of health do not structure these motivations. Instead, they are driven by expansive understandings of health and thriving as linked to families, communities, and lands. In preparing and offering food, they work against the neoliberal framing of what it means to thrive: rather than privileging self-reliance, they promote care for others; rather than focusing on individual responsibility, they imagine and actualize the capacity to thrive as a group commitment; and rather than giving primacy to the idea of self-enhancement, the women in this study explicate how communal support and nourishment are fundamental to well-being.

In relation to fat stem cell science, recall that the use of ADSC therapies or technologies runs the risk of materializing or exacerbating cancer—promoting the thriving of cells toward life in the same moment that they potentially inaugurate the cellular thriving toward death. More broadly, we have outlined how within biocultures of stem cell science, the potential to thrive is viewed as an individual pursuit, a way of optimizing the health of the singular atomized subject who is able to pay for such services. More ethical ways of thriving in relation to fat stem cells are also imaginable, however, but they would rely on first finding ways to mitigate the threat of cancer and would require extensive further investigation as to the broader efficacy of fat stem cell science and therapeutics. If, however, these limitations were overcome, would it not be possible to pursue forms of stem cell altruism rather than harvesting and harnessing these stem cells only for individual use? For instance, if there is so much supposed excess fat, we could conceive of donor services, where those who were interested could gift their fat to others. Along these lines, we could establish fat-banking commons, where gifted fat is stored for communal use—enabling unwanted fat to enter into the circulation of exchange so that those who were in need of ADSCs could access a wider pool of cell reserves. Such possibilities have already been advanced. Indeed, ADSC therapies have been positioned as a potential way to combat rising levels of obesity in the population, with the American Heart Foundation predicting that "future citizens may undergo liposuction to remove excess adipose tissue in 'fat drives'" similar to existing blood drives.[88] To be truly communal, however, such efforts would need to be kept out of the hands of private entities or actors—such as pharmaceutical companies and their investors—who could convert this altruistic gifting into a vehicle of wealth generation: it would require that fat be democratized and made public as a reimagined nonprofit tissue reserve. In each of these scenarios, we see a different understanding of "fat liberation" that works against thinking of fat and health as the property of the individual. And, instead of conceptualizing ADSCs only as the means to optimization, we could conceive of fat stem cells as enabling new forms of ethical conviviality.

If, as we have explored, the dominant affirmation to thrive in relation to fat is regulatory, individualizing, life-threatening, and that which secures inequitable distributions of health, it becomes imperative to find other frames of being, doing, and thriving. Like dominant modes, the alternative versions of thriving that we have outlined here are underscored by a commitment to vitalizing and maintaining sustainable lives. They are distinct, however, in that they share a more expansive understanding of what constitutes life, propose ways to cultivate life that are dispersed across collectives, and advance more socially accountable ways of thriving.

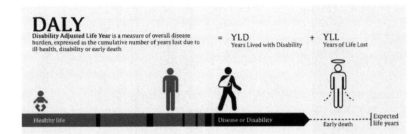

Figure 11. Disability-adjusted life-years (DALY) infographic. Courtesy of Planemad and Radio89. Reproduced under a Creative Commons Attribution-Share Alike 3.0 Unported (CC BY-SA 3.0) license. https://creativecommons.org/licenses/by-sa/3.0/deed.en.

4

Secure

Aging

The biopolitics of security now administers the threshold of life/death: . . . in particular . . . the prolonged forestalling of death.

—Michael Dillon and Luis Lobo-Guerrero,
"Biopolitics of Security in the 21st Century: An Introduction"

The surge of population growth in those aged sixty-five years and older represents "one of the most significant demographic trends in the history of the United States."[1] While this increase in life expectancy might be seen as reason to celebrate, it has also coincided with a rise in the *affirmation to secure the life of the aging subject,* indeed, to secure *against* aging and senescence. The word *security* stems from the Latin *securitas,* deconstructed as *sine curae,* "without troubles or cares." In the context of the aging process, to "secure" refers to safe-guarding, protecting, and fortifying individuals against what are seen as the ravages of old age. Aging/old age has long been associated with burden, pathology, decline, dependency, disability, and potentially living in a state that is death-adjacent. Additionally, as Michel Foucault has argued, aging is equated with the declining productivity of individuals who, "because of their age, fall out of the field of capacity, of activity."[2] Individual declining productivity is, in turn, tethered to ideas of fiscal drain and national decay, as evident in the World Bank's 1994 declaration that a "crisis" in aging "would have a catastrophic effect on productivity growth."[3] As Melinda Cooper has noted, old age is consequently viewed as a wasting or degeneration of productive life.[4] The "problem of old age" is thus a security problematic for biopolitics.[5] In contemporary biocultures of aging, a proliferation of techniques, technologies, and practices seek to promote and regulate life in the face of inevitable senescence; these efforts secure the life of the aging subject and amplify the individual's capacity to live more *and* to age well.[6]

This chapter examines the affirmation to secure found in national and individual efforts to ward against aging in light of biopolitical and disciplinary efforts to maximize "third age." As a descriptor, third age simultaneously denotes a power/knowledge relation, a discourse, and a qualitative rather than chronological "stage of life." The concept of third age was first advanced by Peter Laslett to name a life phase/stage in which older individuals are able to partake in an active, independent, personally fulfilling, healthy life after the constraints of work and child-rearing.[7] Third age only terminates with fourth age, which is marked by deep old age, frailty, and dependence on others. The concept of third age draws on a model first introduced by Robert Havighurst in a 1961 article for the *Gerontologist* and later popularized in the seminal 1987 piece "Human Aging: Usual and Successful" by physician John Rowe and psychologist Robert Kahn. The latter proposed a distinction between "usual" aging (marked by decline and loss) and "successful aging," characterized by avoidance of disease and disability, maintenance of cognitive function, and social engagement.[8] This biomedical-psycho-social model of *aging well* subsequently became a guiding epistemology in gerontology, also appearing under terms such as *productive aging, healthy aging, active aging,* and *vital aging,* among others. Evident not only in biomedicine, this model informs psychological, public health, and general societal narratives around aging. It is central in biocultures of aging: as a discourse, third age/successful aging is "an amalgam of textual and visual messages that appear and circulate in all kinds of public spaces, including but not limited to, the media, policy documents, academic literature, and healthcare organizations."[9]

In the first part of this chapter, we examine various efforts to secure successful aging or "aging well" that, we argue, ostensibly enable individuals to achieve—and maintain themselves within the category of—third age. We specifically focus on the promotion of longevity, independent living, and functional aging—particularly the way these intersect with and condition broader societal understandings of older age and the very experience of aging in U.S. society. Importantly, we show that while these forms of governance pursue the life enhancement of aging subjects, they are regulatory and prescriptive, and they intersect with the governance rationalities of late liberalism. They solidify individualist notions of personhood and emphasize independence and the "need to stay an active producer of a positive health status rather than being a passive consumer of health care."[10]

Within this broader focus on securing aging well, we shift to analyzing biofinancial security mechanisms, namely, metrics associated with global health economics that have been adopted in the United States. Such metrics are used to assess the health and age-impaired states of the population as scientific and economic "problems," to identify where funding should be directed, what health interventions should be made, and how resources should be allocated. The accompanying health economic strategies seek to preempt the economic burden of an aging population—to secure against decline and old age. However, we argue that, similar to the promotion of third age, the biofinancialization of aging populations seemingly suggests the maintenance of life but in fact exacts costs that imperil lives.

In the second part of the chapter, we consider how decline is governed. Specifically, we focus on the biomedical promotion of "more life at any cost" for those who can be said to be on the brink of fourth age. Looking to the range of biomedical interventions that seek to secure the lives of ailing older individuals, we examine how dominant logics of biocultures of aging structure understandings of "what should be done" for those nearing death and the implications of the affirmation to secure in ever-later and deep old age. Following this, we address the "biomedical aftermath"—how the affirmation to secure aging subjects within the biomedical arena is conditioned by practices of "deadly care" within the broader political economy of institutionalizing elders in the United States. We explore how these factors actually delimit caring for those in age-related decline within the biomedical sphere and relegate infirm older individuals to nursing homes and hospice care. Here we consider how such sites function as the "shadowlands" of aging and actually work against the "make live" principle of biopolitics. Concluding the chapter, we ask, what alternative biocultures of aging might exist or be imagined to reaffirm aging based on more positive understandings of dependency in older age, interrelatedness between the aged and other members of society, and vulnerability?

Securing "Aging Well"

A paradoxical discourse of aging as both burden and opportunity dominates policy and public culture. With projections of the number of Americans aged sixty-five and older to double by 2030, policies aimed at the problems of aging at the population level couch health in economic terms and entreat individuals to manage their own existences.[11] Third age discourse emphasizes new consumer markets and the "active effort of individuals to shape their experience of ageing in such a way that it reduces demands or dependency upon public systems of provision."[12] Biocultures of aging thus entail a variety of mechanisms that "secure life"—against aging, decline, and unproductivity—and enlist new forms of governance concerning how to age well. We examine here a few key everyday forms of governmentality that support third age discourse and secure aging: first, the interrelated promotion of longevity, independent living, and functional aging, and second, biofinancializing old age—reducing life to a funding problem through complex economic thinking—to secure against the cost of old age. While by no means an exhaustive account of the dynamic biocultural arena of aging, these cases map what kinds of aging are encouraged, how that aging is organized, and the limitations and dangers of this governing.[13]

Longevity, Independent Living, and Functional Aging

The pursuit of longevity is central to the discourse of third age and entails securing the productivity of aging. By maintaining productivity in various forms and expressions, the idea is that people will live longer and healthier lives: they will age well and enjoy finer lives. While the goal of making people live longer and age better is clearly laudable and not one that should be dismissed, the way that longevity is defined and pursued can be highly disciplinary and often detrimental to the elderly and anyone aging more broadly—with particularly deleterious consequences for people whose lives do not align with normative expectations of independence, agency, bodily autonomy, and constant activity.[14]

In U.S. biocultures of aging, bodies are disciplined to manage aging through activities that secure dependency-free life expectancy.[15] Sharon R. Kaufman explains: "the activities that constitute longevity making, like so many other socio-medical practices, constitute a site for the governing of life and the emergence of new forms of ethical comportment and social participation. Those activities . . . also lie at the heart of debates about health care rationing and reform."[16] In other words, longevity is not merely an innocent quest for "more life": it is a normative project of not being a burden on society and securing productivity through reflexive, often obligatory self-care practices. Older people are encouraged to be active, mobile, autonomous, experimental, networked, and consumer oriented—with the goals of wellness and visible inclusion in public life.[17] Courtney Everts Mykytyn characterizes this as "a push to infuse popular representations and experiences of aging with notions of creativity, leisure, wisdom, and productivity . . . which create[s] a moral imperative for older individuals to both remain engaged and contribute to society."[18] Lifelong learning opportunities (online professional programs, university extension courses, etc.) are seen as an economic imperative and opportunity to meet the developmental needs of older people through intellectual and creative engagement. Senior employment and volunteer work additionally support the idea that middle age and up is a time for self-discovery and productivity. For example, Encore.org, an online platform for redirecting the skills and experience of those in midlife toward "second acts for the greater good," challenges the idea that aging is a problem by advancing a new narrative for later life as "encore life"—characterized by individual renewal and social impact.[19] Another organization, ReServe, advertises the goal of establishing one hundred thousand "reservists" by 2030, referring to individuals over fifty-five that the organization matches with nonprofits to help social causes.[20]

Many of these programs understand successful aging to be an *ongoing achievement of the self*—as a project of discovery and well-being—that involves the active consumption of health care and maintaining one's productivity and personhood until the moment of death.[21] While these are admirable goals that can benefit one's physical health, "activity" serves as a panacea for political problems mounted by state disinvestment in health care, pensions, and other entitlements for the elderly. As the population grows old, successful aging means "being a busy body."[22] Longevity effectively becomes an ideological project of securing a lifelong state of consumer-oriented adulthood through self-responsibility and virtuous activity. Regardless of the personal feelings of an older person toward her work or voluntary contributions to society, seniors are interpellated in an ageist culture that positions them as a burden on society. Moreover, the volunteer economy of the elderly rests on class position: many Americans have or can expect little to no retirement; retirement has become a privilege rather than a basic right of old age. Senior volunteering and encore careers may not be within reach for people who must work longer before retiring— or cannot retire—and who take on expanding responsibilities for informal care work, particularly women. There are also ethical and equity concerns about enlisting seniors in auxiliary support services for an increasingly gutted public sector.

Independent living is also a key component of third age discourse. In the broadest sense, the goal of independent living is tethered to basic ideas about what it means to be an individual—such as the ability to be autonomous and capable of directing your own life. In the spirit of such ideas, and especially for financially mobile and retirement-abled persons, an aggressive entrepreneurial "Aging 2.0" urban market promotes senior lifestyles, housing, medical care, everyday products, and financial goods that allegedly secure independent lifestyles. Campaigns about "aging in place," in particular, promise longevity and autonomy linked to location and remaining at home, tying successful aging to livability indices and urban metrics.[23] For example, "Best Cities for Successful Aging" rankings assess how metropolitan areas "enable people to age independently and productively, with security and good health," using a "livability" rubric that includes community engagement and wellness, coordinated with health care access, educational and financial opportunities, transportation, and convenience.[24] An expanding industry of smart home technologies advertises dependency-free adult living—with the competence and fitness to conduct daily life. Intelligent homes equipped with wireless communications, infotechnologies, and infrastructural features geared to the aging promise independence by converting domestic space into health-monitoring and caregiving spaces.[25] Historically, home health care has entailed nurses and caregivers traveling to a patient's home several times a week for monitoring and treatment, but smart home technology supports varying degrees of "telecare," such as long-distance monitoring of patient blood pressure, heart rate, and other vital signs and remote communication with health providers and family/community caregivers. Remote care might entail body-worn sensors that measure health data, monitoring systems that manage physiological data and activities in the home, and/or varying levels of medical emergency response and fall detection.[26]

Advocates of telecare/telehealth contend that such technologies "will reduce hospital readmission, give patients greater independence, and improve health, by allowing senior citizens to live at home longer prior to or instead of requiring nursing home care."[27] The combination of smart home with remote care invites the biomedical gaze within the home and body in new and intensified ways via myriad sensors and other ambient assisted living technologies. Stealth Health, for instance, claims that "high-fidelity data" are gathered and analyzed continuously via hidden sensors that "monitor the human body from a distance, never making contact and without maintenance."[28] Everyday home furnishings and appliances have been developed with motion sensors, digital radars, video monitoring, and temperature and light sensors to assess health and wellness. Blankets with vital signs sensors track how one sleeps; carpets with RFID technology monitor motion in the home environment to secure an established routine. Still other home technologies promise independent living through mobile technologies and social media applications that medicalize routine activities and coordinate companionship with medical compliance. For example, Reminder Rosie is a personalized, voice-controlled reminder system designed to assist older adults with memory loss. Equipped with a hands-free "senior-friendly clock interface," the system sends reminders about medications, appointments, and everyday tasks to "maximize independence, provide personalized care, relieve caregiver stress, [and] sustain medical adherence."[29] Products such as Pill Pets dispense medication through home companion robots, endeavoring to foster obedience and medical adherence through the emotional bond between the aging person and a pet.[30] The care coach service GeriJoy organizes caregiving companionship—when family, friends, or local caregivers are not around—through a tablet interface connected 24/7 to "a remote team of human caregivers and advanced computer intelligence systems."[31]

These technologies assist in the governance of the way older people live: they expand and both qualify and limit care, produce new risks, intensify individual responsibility for managing one's own end of life, and open up new kinds of surveillance of everyday embodied experience. This biomedicalization of daily living reveals that "the boundaries between coercion and consent begin to blur as new administrative technologies promote autonomy, informed choice, and non-directiveness within a general ethos of 'quality of life.'"[32] Quality of life and independent living are achieved through home surveillance and paternalistic biomedical penetrations of home space and the body that impose limitations on the civil liberties of the elderly at home—an attenuated form of independence and *insecure* senior citizenship. The Fourth Amendment right to privacy, in particular, is at risk: the privacy rule to protect health information—under the Health Insurance Portability and Accountability Act (HIPAA)—likely does not cover health information and biological metrics collected and transmitted through mobile technologies or third parties that monitor homes. The monitoring of activities of daily living (ADLs), such as how often you turn on the television or visit the toilet, does not necessarily meet the definition of health data and is therefore outside the purview of privacy protection. Because aging at home involves relinquishing some degree of autonomy and privacy rights, it may lead to a general condition of "house arrest" for seniors and data-mining operations.[33]

Moreover, home technologies and aging at home remain inaccessible to many people; government subsidies are restricted or nonexistent. On a basic economic level, home care invites you to live in your house longer, equipped with technologies that assist you, but you must also manage your own end of life with fewer public resources and potentially no retirement or personal savings or community around you. The adjustment to old age takes the form of an individual ethical domain and enterprise that exacerbates rather than remedies structural inequities and differences in old age based on class, race, gender, and so forth. Old people are governed within lifestyle profiles allied with neoliberal agendas that vilify dependency and treat "aging bodies and identities as risky, vulnerable, and in need of self-vigilance."[34] Just as approaches to gerontology and health promotion programs emphasize mobility, cognition, and social activities, successful aging in the home is inherently normative and restrictive, offering blueprints for healthy aging tethered to middle-class moral and family-oriented conventions.[35] Home care, in this sense, may intensify moral regulation of aging—that is, aging becomes a kind of work ethic or even workfare that is the responsibility of every individual.[36] Moreover, the notion of "independence" that provides the rationale for the expanding senior tech market *secures against* the leaky, unstable embodied reality of aging. Independent living and successful aging tend to be anti-aging, prophylactic discourses that shut down the opportunity to come to terms with the relentless coming-together and coming-apart of the messy existence of older persons, with their assistive devices, home monitoring, Medicare/Medicaid restrictions, and vulnerable shifting bodies.

Underwriting the ideological projects of longevity and independent living, *third age discourse promotes the logic of "functional aging"* and extends this across the whole of life, demarcating an ever-expanding zone of governance: of midlife, prime life, and extended adulthood. Functionality, as a concept, is tied to the idea that the body should operate according to normative criteria of and for embodiment: this is inextricable from the Cartesian notion that the body is subservient to the mind—that the self has a body that it controls. In a narrower sense, and in relation to our focus here, to be functional (to have a body that works properly) requires fitness, enablement, avoidance of impairment, and prevention of disease.

We see increased emphasis on functionality in the fact that one cannot officially die of old age in the United States—it is not a specific enough reason for dying to be included in the standard list of contributing and underlying causes of death used by state and federal agencies.[37] Instead, aging—

unmoored from the idea of a natural life course—is treated like a disease and subject to intervention.[38] Functional age—the idea that age can and should be defined in terms of functional capacity—"drives the imperative to biologize the aging process apart from chronological aging by co-ordinating the body's biomarkers."[39] These biomarkers of aging—specific to individuals and even differentiated by tissues, organs, or organ systems within the same body or organism—can be measured and predicted, thus allowing for customized intervention and alteration of rates of aging. "Exhaustive batteries of tests, aggregations of data, scales, indices and self-reports" based on these biomarkers implicate the individual as an active participant in striving toward functionality and the "collective ideal of enabled fitness."[40] Stephen Katz and Barbara L. Marshall characterize this now-dominant bioculture of aging: "the biosocial rationalities of functional age and independent living correspond, therefore, linking functional bodies to functional populations. Supporting this correspondence are the bio-identities by which people can know themselves as functional and participate in a gerontological culture of enablement."[41]

Quantifiable standards of functionality circulate well beyond eldercare under the signs of what is normal, natural, and healthy. The goal of being functional connects with broader social mandates around active and mobile lifestyles, responsible self-care, adaptability, freedom of choice, and economic independence.[42] The objective of functionality enables pharmacological and therapeutic interventions into *aging at any age* to preempt or modify dysfunctions, pathologies, or potential disease. This stretching of midlife to late life makes the risks of old age more present in midlife; simultaneously, "with midlife the universal ideal, older people meet the stringent criteria of successful aging only insofar as they are not 'old.'"[43] At increasingly younger ages, people are exhorted to monitor their lifestyles and modify their behaviors throughout life—avoiding disease and disability, maintaining high physical and cognitive functional capacity, and actively engaging in life—to ward off midlife decline.[44] One example is the idea of "retirement readiness" or "retirement fitness," along with the midlife popularity of activity trackers such as the Fitbit or Oura ring.[45]

Biomedicine also promises to secure against bodily decline through biological preemption and emancipation.[46] This signals the genetic determination of life-span and the increased significance of gathering health intelligence through the biosurveillance of risk. Human longevity entails "cracking the code" of the body as a data machine, to prevent disease;

this essentially molecularizes healthy aging—that is, it biologizes securing against aging.[47] The company Human Longevity Inc. exemplifies the bio-social rationalities behind this reliance on informational technologies that connect individuals and groups to genetic datspheres and their experts. Billed as "your health intelligence partner," Human Longevity claims to be "revolutionizing human health by generating more data and deeper understanding into what can keep you living healthier longer."[48] Its products include HLIQ Whole Genome, "a comprehensive report ordered by your physician that compares every letter of your DNA with the world's largest database of sequenced genomes and phenotype data, to reveal your best opportunities for proactive, preventative health planning."[49] Framing genetic research and testing as an investment in oneself—"Health is the new wealth. Invest in yours."—the company enlists participants to biosecuritize the self against the body/biology (in terms of disease, decline, aging, death) and contribute to a heroic culture of perfectability and bio-investments in longevity.

The capacity of individuals to pursue such data-driven strategies to preempt disease and decline again depends heavily on a basic foundation that many people lack in the United States: "adequate income, access to affordable and nutritional food, a healthy and safe neighborhood in which to live, and affordable, good-quality health care."[50] Additionally, as Katz and Marshall explain, "health literacy is embedded in class, gender, racial and regional inequalities and hierarchical forms of cultural capital."[51] Understanding aging merely as market trend or genomic sequence obscures how the population of older people experiences aging as a diverse process along heterogeneous axes of difference with uneven access to health and wellness resources.[52] The emphasis placed on individual management of aging in late liberalism fails to address the structural aspects of unevenly distributed life-spans and premature deaths—which continue apace regardless of biomedical advancements in longevity. An emphasis on "exceptionalism" in health and productive aging—"I made it; why can't you?"—does nothing to eliminate larger patterns of oppression.[53] If you are unsuccessful, it is your failure, not society's.

Moreover, the pursuit of functionality, as it intersects with notions of longevity and independent living, bolsters "cultural denial of disability, dependency, and ultimately death."[54] Disability is particularly repudiated. Supplanting an earlier dread of aging with a more specific fear of aging with a disability, norms of positive aging treat visible "oldness" as disability and consider disability to be a reflection of failure. This galvanizes fears of bodily suffering and even of the elderly themselves, leading to inadequate policy responses because people whose bodies evoke suffering or are "out of control" are blamed; "older people with functional limitations, most of whom are women, [are denied] the dignity of their struggle to accept what they cannot change."[55] Equating good health with successful aging—and disability and poor health with failure—ignores the diverse ways that individuals experience aging physiologically, emotionally, and socially.[56] The notion of productive aging is essentially anti-aging, in that one learns nothing about what it means to experience "becoming spent" through the passage of time.[57] Instead of fostering a sense of accomplishment and commitment to the meaningfulness of aging as a kind of transformation connected to and preceding death, longevity strategies reduce aging to the most basic norms, devalue old age, and desocialize death.[58] Brett Nielson warns, "At stake is nothing less than a rethinking of models of citizenship and economy that presuppose able-bodied subjectivity, a proviso that applies as much to celebratory notions of the Third Age that suppress the knowledge of eventual bodily breakdown, as to the normative concepts of well-being and human capability that derive from the body-related universalisms of Western thought."[59]

Biofinancializing Old Age

The pursuit of active, independent living and other strategies that forestall decline are mechanisms that aim to secure a population that "ages well." Third age discourse and the "longevity revolution" of delaying aging aim to keep people healthier to live better lives *and* preempt the burden of aging on society. Advocacy for the future health and economic value of older Americans, however, confronts the social implications and political–economic consequences of expected longer life-spans—and, specifically, the onslaught of baby boomers approaching middle and later ages and the looming problem of Social Security shortfalls and rising medical demands. The political rhetoric on aging at national and international levels warns against a "global aging crisis," "age bomb," and "baby boomer bust." In this context, new metrics associated with global health economics have arisen to construct and assess the health of the population as a scientific and economic problem. Institutions and individuals have adopted such quantitative biofinancial techniques to secure against the threat of old age: the tools highlight areas of concern and stress points in the population's health and conditions of aging where public campaigns and interventions can be made and where individuals can focus to change their lives. While third age pursuits of longevity, independent living, and maintaining functionality seek to preempt the burden of aging, health economic strategies *secure against decline through the biofinancialization of old age*—within the context of both a neoliberal environment of devolving age-care services and the transferring of responsibility for the maintenance of the elderly to communities, networks of social capital, and markets. The biofinancializing of old age, we argue, positions aging as a security problematic for biopolitics via framing and assessing the burden of aging in terms of economic loss and costs.[60]

A neoliberal global health regime has tied the management of human bodies closely to economic management, with cost-effectiveness the method for prioritizing health services.[61] While the field of global health is expansive and international, the older/aging population of a nation is perceived as a threat, and thus governance aims to secure against the decline of the national body. The burden of old age is defined here not as genetic or eugenic but rather as the costs borne by national medical/health care systems. In an aging U.S. society, "a growing array of life-extending medical interventions, Medicare policy and an ethic of individual decision-making together contribute to the deepening societal tension between controlling health care costs and enabling health consumer use of life-sustaining technologies."[62] Measuring aggregated health allows for prioritizing specific applications of health care funds and assessing their success. Instead of mapping disease patterns and scrutinizing the problem of morbidity in relation to deaths, biopolitical governance focuses here on calculating disease burdens and examining "morbid living"—that is, the functional and impaired health states of the population and the health-spans (not life-spans) of individuals. Part of the late twentieth-century influx of rating scales, scoring systems, and various indices assessing quality of life and well-being, measurements such as "years of potential life lost" (YPLL) make nonfatal outcomes calculable. Similarly, "health-adjusted life-years" (HALY), "disability-adjusted life-years" (DALY), and "quality-adjusted life-years" (QALY) perform a new epistemology: departing from measuring life/death rates of a population, these metrics support health status valuations, quality of life scores, and calculations of morbid living based on severity, disability, impairment, and functional aging.[63] The focus on decline connects lost life chances and suffering with the costs to society—whether direct costs to health care or indirect costs of lost productivity.[64] Experts in this area account for loss of healthy life due to disease, death, and disability on a national competitiveness and global scale. The data are used to redesign and optimize health systems according to the logic of economic maximization—investing in health as an economic project and economizing life by imagining health as a form of human capital.[65] This approach weds life expectancy to productivity—the impetus of the discourse of third age.

The health metric DALY, for example, measures disease burden at the population level in terms of the "reduction of the functioning capacity of individuals, defined as the 'ability to perform ADLs such as learning, working, feeding and clothing oneself.'"[66] From the 1990s on, DALY has been used as a way to assist governments in setting health priorities. In one of its prominent appearances, the *Lancet* in 2012 published DALY for 291 diseases and injuries in twenty-one regions on the global burden of disease from 1990 to 2010.[67] The work accounted for population health by calculating the incidence of health and disease at a global aggregate level. Previously, mortality statistics and risk of death were used to calculate the number of deaths from disease; DALY, by contrast, factors in loss of healthy life due to disease, disability, and death by measuring mortality and morbidity together in the same unit of analysis. The overall "problem space" of DALY is the loss of the mode of life proper to competitiveness as a consequence of the impact of disease on the individual and collective. DALY's underlying claim is that the impact of a disease or condition may not be fatal, but its disabling effects contribute to economic losses, diminished productivity, and strain on health systems.[68] DALY essentially offers an approach to individual and societal worth that synthesizes biology and economy: it considers health in relation to economic contribution, attempts to quantify it, and then uses the figure to evaluate economic and thus social contribution.

DALY accomplishes this "economization of life by disaggregating lifetimes into component units of time and reassembling life as a revenue stream [as human capital] to be maximized through practices of self-investment in one's own health."[69] Whereas vital statistics previously measured life as a coherent unity from birth to death, DALY measures loss of life as the loss of its constituent parcels of time.[70] Put differently, DALY negatively measures the severity of disability caused by disease, decline, aging, and so on, multiplied by the duration anticipated until remission or death. One DALY is one year of healthy life lost to premature death or fractionally to disease and disability, following the equation DALYs = YLL (years of life lost) + YDL (years lived with a disability of specific duration and severity). The calculation gauges the loss of health from an imagined ideal state, in terms of the present value of the future impact of life lost to death and disease. Following the economic convention of prioritizing immediate over future gains by discounting the future at a steady rate, DALY is a decremental measure, meaning the value of years of life lost decreases as you get older. In other words, the equation discounts the value of years of life as one ages; it also equates aging with disability and disability with decline. In application, DALY serves as a forecasting technique that attempts to optimize rates on returns of investment in health; the metric facilitates the use of cost–benefit analysis in prioritizing potential health interventions in the units of dollars spent per DALY gained.

DALY and other like metrics support a market-led biopolitical regime by ascribing a value of life that, as Emma Whyte Laurie argues, leads to "the *de*valuation of certain populations," specifically the elderly.[71] Kevin Morgan contends that any method of valuing human life for planning purposes inherently discriminates against older people; any allocation of resources on the basis of age risks moving, in David C. Thomasma's words, "the elderly into the house of the dead, precisely because they 'cut off' the elderly from the modes of care we offer to other persons in society."[72] DALY calculations are open to misuse as a means of channeling resources away from the elderly and chronically sick due to the economic rationality that undergirds the metrics. The underlying logic of efficient and cost-effective resource allocation places limits on the availability of health care in response to background conditions of scarcity and austerity. These limits are perceived to be apolitical and neutral—achieved through technical methodologies and instruments. Yet, as numerous critics have noted, the utilitarian technocratic approach is incapable of addressing distributional issues: efficiency supersedes equity and can be (or is) used to exclude parts of the population under the banner of "what's best for society."[73]

In this respect, DALY simultaneously exacerbates and obscures inequitable distributions of life and resources by setting a standard of life expectancy that decontextualizes calculations of the global burden of disease (measured in DALYs) from actual health conditions of people. An ideal life expectancy is assumed to be the same across the population, with no acknowledgment of highly variable sociocultural and historical conditions, removing any geography and material conditions that define or limit life:

the limit to life is relocated to a speculative future where it serves as the point at which death is no longer premature. Furthermore, by recasting health as human capital—an investment commodity representing the total amount of time for market and nonmarket activities—the biofinancializing of old age sorts out high-mortality populations as failed investments and may justify a neoliberal biopolitics of disposability—the abandonment of parts of the population—based on projected losses.[74] An individual may experience this as a kind of double jeopardy in an unjust distributive political economy of resources and care: after a disaster strikes a patient and leaves them with a poor quality of life, such metrics could disqualify them for life-saving treatment because of preexisting conditions and relegate them to a socially acceptable *minimum* of care via an expanding sector of hospices for the chronically sick in addition to the terminally ill.[75]

While DALY rationalizes the *discounting of elderly lives* via assigning different values to years of life lost at different stages of life (an elder is less valued than a middle-aged person, who is considered to belong to the most productive part of society), it is disability that is cast as the ultimate unproductive life, due to the weighting of disability severity within DALY calculations. Using S. Lochlann Jain's term, DALY's weighing of states of compromised health has a "mortality effect": the discounting of the lives of disabled people who are relegated in some applications of DALY to a status worse than death.[76] Disability is considered to undermine economic productivity potential—part of a broader imaginary of disability as a life without a future unless capacitated through biomedical and/or biocapitalist futures that "overcome" disability.[77] The metric basically channels embodied vulnerabilities that stem from social relations of class, race, gender, sexuality, age, and so on—any social, political, and economic conditions that delimit reproductive futurity and life expectancy—into the category of disability, as an expansive, flexible area marked for disinvestment. The elderly and those who do not age well are at risk of being punished for conditions beyond their control via the market logics of a utilitarian health economics.

Governing in Decline

The governance of aging, as we have explored, works to secure "aging well" by maximizing third age—by promoting longevity, independent living, and functionality. At the same time, the biofinancialization of old age and the techniques and metrics that are used to assess the burden of what is seen as "age-related decline" are deployed to secure against the costs of aging populations. In what follows, we consider *how age-related decline itself is governed,* that is, how the administration or management of aging stretches into what might be termed "later life"—into the last moments of life itself. Here the dominant logics of biocultures of aging structure expectations of what should be done for and to the elderly. We examine two key areas of the governing of age-related decline: first, we consider what is often the relentless effort to secure the lives of ailing older individuals on the brink of fourth age within the biomedical arena. We ask, what are the limitations and costs (social, personal, conceptual) of such efforts? Second, we explore the broader political economy of eldercare in the United States to analyze how economic rationalities condition the treatment of older individuals both in hospital care and in the biomedical aftermath—specifically in the extrabiomedical environments of nursing homes and hospice care. We argue that, rather than securing the lives of those on the event horizon of life, these extrabiomedical sites can be considered "shadowlands," where those in fourth age are subject to forms of "deadly care" and are often abandoned.

More Life at Any Cost?

The biomedical arena is a key site where the affirmation to secure aging subjects emerges, precisely because biomedicine "exists in a cultural milieu that stresses longevity by any means and at any cost."[78] Within this context, seriously ill older individuals are increasingly encouraged to push against the risk of death—to avoid death a little longer—in order to gain additional years, months, weeks, or simply days. This effort to secure more life is enabled through increased biomedical interventions in later life. Indeed, the biomedical model of health—which focuses on biological factors of health promotion, generally to the exclusion of psychological, environmental, and social influences—undergirds this life-making: it is viewed as "the right (and perhaps only) tool for managing the problems of aging."[79] Thus these "problems" are supposedly "solved" through the consumption or purchase of more and more high-cost medical services and technologies by those who are able to do so. Reflecting a lack of steadfast clinical assumptions about what can be done for older patients, individuals in their seventies, eighties, and even nineties are now undergoing, often as a matter of course, procedures such as cardiac bypass, angioplasty, stent, and pacemaker placement, renal dialysis, kidney transplant, and aggressive cancer treatments to extend their lives. What this highlights, as critical gerontologists and scholars of aging have noted, is that chronological age is receding as a factor in treatment.[80] That is to say, for physicians in particular, the age of a patient is no longer a predictor of whether a particular procedure is viewed as warranted. Instead, "clinical responsibility means performing life-extending procedures regardless of age, as long as there is a *possibility* that *potential* benefits *might* outweigh the risks."[81]

Interventions such as those noted above have become routinized, normalized, and expected, as Sharon Kaufman and Lakshmi Fjord have stated, "regardless of end-stage medical conditions . . . and irrespective of financial burden to families or social costs to the nation." This, they argue, is a particularly U.S. phenomenon, "in which progress and individual aspiration are manifest in technological know-how and technical solutions."[82] Importantly, it is also the very routinization of treatment that rules the choices that both clinicians and patients make. On the clinical side, as any given (and approved) technology emerges, clinicians are guided to think of it as an "ethical necessity."[83] Treatment becomes an imperative precisely because of "technical ability" (that is, when a technique has been perfected and proven to be potentially efficacious) and because the patient meets the criteria for intervention. On the patient side, individuals and their families experience the *imperative to treat* "as hope materialized and actualized."[84] The routinization of treatment also produces a form of moral obligation for individuals and their families: faced with the choice of life-extending treatment, they must take on the responsibility of balancing too much or too little intervention. The conjuncture of ethical necessity/moral obligation and technological capacity both shapes "what should be done" in terms of treating older patients and functions as a form of governance—regulating both vital materiality and how disease or decline is encountered.

Cardiac care treatment offers a salient case in point. Life-prolonging cardiac treatments—which include angioplasty stents, coronary bypass graft surgery (CABG), and implantable cardiovascular defibrillators (ICDs)—are now becoming routine in the United States for those in their eighth, ninth, and even tenth decades. This expansion of cardiac treatment is in part due to the proliferation of risk discourse: the idea that risk is everywhere and should be monitored and then intervened upon.[85] In terms of ICDs in particular, it is risk that is now treated.[86] We see this in the criteria for ICD implantation and classifications for eligibility for Medicare reimbursement for this procedure: before 2003, ICDs would only be implanted and eligible for reimbursement under Medicare if a patient presented with a minimum of one incident of cardiac arrest or documented arrhythmia; in 2003, eligibility criteria to receive both the device and reimbursement changed, expanding to include those who had had one heart attack or who met certain measures of declining heart function.[87] By 2006, however, ICD treatment and Medicare coverage were broadened to most individuals with weakened hearts, even if they had not had a cardiac event.[88] This wider casting of the net of who can and should receive ICDs highlights that the device is now conceptualized as a safety net or prophylaxis. It is used simply because of the existence of risk (to prevent the possibility of future heart attack), not because of the existence of disease or symptoms. It operates, then, as a measure of biopolitical risk management for those demarcated as belonging to a high-risk group. At the same time, the risk *produced* as a by-product of treatment is seen to have decreasing relevance as ICDs become standard. And, precisely because they have become so common, they are difficult for patients to refuse, even if the benefits are negligible.

The risk discourse that dictates cardiac and other forms of biomedical care in the elderly "often provides the rationale for intensifying the frequency and aggressiveness of treatments," producing what Janet K. Shim, Ann J. Russ, and Sharon R. Kaufman call "technological incrementalism."[89] They explain this as a process in which increasingly normalized noninvasive treatments become the grounds for justifying ever more subsequent and invasive interventions. What we see, then, is an "interventional continuum" or intervention spiral, where elderly patients receive more and more extreme supports or technological aides in order to secure/prolong life: an ICD, a series of stents, multiple invasive heart surgeries, an oxygen tank, a permanent catheter, and so forth. The paradoxes at work here are that the aged body is simultaneously viewed as diseased and a space for intervention, and age is viewed as irrelevant for medical intervention in one and the same moment that an age focus (to push back decline) permeates biomedicine.

Importantly, increased biomedical interventions in later life—the seemingly relentless effort to secure life in older individuals—often create a denial of death: *everything* is done to deny death and there is often a lack of acknowledgment of death as a possible outcome until all treatments have been tried.[90] Two key effects can be noted here. First, the kinds of biomedical interventions we have named can prolong life into *morbid life* (this is, needless to say, another paradox). Morbid life can be defined as a long process of dying, where death or deathlike existence is brought into life.

Put another way, this might be thought of as death by degrees, what critical gerontologist Harry Moody calls "prolonged morbidity" and what Sara Manning Peskin names "protracted dying."[91] We might also consider this form of death-in-life as prosthetic or attenuated life, where life's continuance is only enabled through the disciplining of the individual body, where the body is hooked up to or intervened upon by various forms of biomedical technologies and techniques—sustained by machines and devices. Second, the incrementalism of these biomedical interventions can rule out the possibility of what is thought of as a "good death." Recall that the affirmation to secure life/health operates through the promotion of responsibilized and entrepreneurial activity, which is equated with autonomy/independence: this is considered the "good life" in biocultures of aging, and it is this good life that supposedly leads to or enables the "good death"—which is also valorized as autonomous (crafted through a series of individual choices) and without burdensome pain, symptoms, and technological dependence. Additionally, the good death relies on the biomedical concept of the compression of morbidity: to "compress the time horizon between the onset of chronic illness or disability and the time in which a person dies."[92] Yet such a situation is at best constrained or at worst foreclosed. Pain, symptoms, and technology are now part and parcel of the march toward death due to the normalization of biomedical interventions in eldercare. Rather than compressing morbidity, these interventions, as we have noted, often prolong morbid conditions in life. Given that 63 percent of Americans die in hospitals, autonomy is severely limited in death: the trajectories of dying and death itself are intimately administered through hospital regulations and health structures.[93]

The Biomedical Aftermath: Shadowlands of Dependency

The curative imperative of biomedicine and the affirmation to secure aging subjects are further complicated by the political economy of eldercare in the United States. Most specifically, neoliberal rationalities—the market logics that have increasingly been applied to the delivery of treatment—are restructuring the care of older individuals. Such restructuring is evident, for instance, in what is known as the Diagnosis-related Group (DRG) Prospective Payment System. Introduced in 1983 by Medicare, the DRG system is a method of prospective (rather than retroactive) reimbursement by Medicare made to a hospital based on a patient's initial diagnosis. A patient must fit into one diagnosis-related group (originally of 468 categories), and each individual DRG has a predetermined fixed price attached to it, based on the average cost per case for that category.[94] This accounting technology is "thought to contain within it specific incentives to motivate hospitals to control costs of treatment to Medicare beneficiaries."[95] The focus is *economic efficiency*—a boon to the administration of recording, analyzing, and allocating costs of individual patient services (e.g., medications, procedures, tests, room and board) in line with the prices set for a particular DRG.

However, given that Medicare provides health insurance mainly for Americans over sixty-five years old, the consequences of this desired economic efficiency predominantly affect the elderly. Hospitals have been known to concentrate on what are considered the most lucrative DRGs (also referred to as "product lines") because they have been compelled by the system to reassess procedures where cost exceeds revenue. This has also led to what is known as DRG "dumping"—where nonprofitable DRGs and patients are rejected from other hospitals and dumped in city-run or state hospitals—resulting in the redistribution and rationing of care. Moreover, to control costs within the pre-set price, hospital managers often push doctors to treat patients for less (by ordering fewer tests and discharging early), meaning that patients are generally now discharged "quicker and sicker."[96] Ultimately, the DRG system has changed the patient experience of care, as Alistair M. Preston has noted: the disease category rather than the patient is the focus, and the imperatives of the system "heighten the economic dimensions of important treatment and leave less room for the human dimension of care."[97]

The huge expansion of the for-profit sector in the U.S. biomedical sphere—where the provision of health services has increasingly come to be viewed as a business—is another factor that has led to the restructuring of eldercare. This is especially evident in the rise of for-profit investor-owned hospitals. For example, between 1975 and 1983, investor-owners added five hundred new hospitals and sixty-two thousand beds to the health market, more than doubling holdings during this period.[98] The sphere has also seen a massive expansion of investor-owned companies ("systems" within which one company will have multiple holdings), leading to a shrinking of health care market diversity. The objective here is primarily *profit maximization* for shareholders rather than care delivery, a scenario that has specific effects on services aimed at the elderly. In a hospital context where the average number of days of stay in acute care has plummeted to fewer than five—as a means of controlling costs and maximizing profits—elderly patients are particularly subject to precarity, due to their more frail health and recovery capacities after discharge.[99]

Additional changes to eldercare delivery have occurred due to the rise in investor-owned ambulatory care facilities, such as outpatient surgery, urgent care centers, dialysis clinics, cardiac rehabilitation centers, physical rehabilitation centers, and diagnostic imaging/radiology centers that have proliferated with the marketization of U.S. health care. These ambulatory services are often "multiproducts" owned by hospitals (that then enable or create a stream in and out of hospital), where for-profit status is dominant.[100] The consequences for the elderly of this rise in ambulatory services are numerous: they now often see multiple doctors who do not necessarily cross-communicate, meaning that care can be compromised; elderly ambulatory care patients may have inadequate knowledge about their current therapies—due to the fracturing of health care, advancing age, and often cognitive decline—which can negatively affect health; and the increase in health care costs associated with ambulatory care directly impacts the elderly, who generally have lower incomes and greater health needs.[101] These examples highlight that hospitals and satellite health services are increasingly governed by profit imperatives, efficiency, and cost accountancy (especially linked to cost reimbursement from government). Such rationales create a situation in which any form of dependency is disavowed in the biomedical arena, and long-term care for the elderly is foreclosed.[102]

Sustained care for dependent older individuals instead takes place largely outside the immediate biomedical arena: it is the extrabiomedical sphere that ostensibly secures lives in decline. What we see, however, is that older frail individuals—in fourth age—are often channeled into a range of *shadowlands*—landscapes of abandonment—where they are made invisible and subject to discursive erasure at the event horizon of life. This erasure is in part produced by the biomedical model, which pushes mortality to the perimeters of social consciousness. Nursing homes and hospices are two such shadowlands or biocultural spheres of erasure that might be said to produce a form of "social death."[103] They both physically sequester the ill and dying, out of sight from the general populace (often in banal/ordinary landscapes in plain sight); they are socially alienating to residents, who are excluded from the lives they have led; and they both often negate the subjectivity of individuals in their care, in that the needs and agency of the elderly are often subsumed in the very process—and proceduralization—of delivering "eldercare."

Nursing homes, for example, broadly exist to provide care to dependent elderly individuals who can no longer look after themselves due to physical and/or cognitive impairment—those subjects Nancy Ettlinger names the "infirm elderly."[104] These institutions deliver round-the-clock medical attention and assist residents in navigating their ADLs, such as bathing, dressing, toileting, and eating. Nursing homes can provide short-term care, often following hospitalization, and/or long-term care for those who are no longer able to return to or remain in their homes. This care is publicly funded for individuals who do not privately cover their costs, with Medicare providing higher-paying reimbursement for short-term stays and Medicaid funding long-term care. In that nursing homes administer the social problem of infirmity in old age, they can be viewed as biopolitical institutions that foster and maintain the "end of life"—by securing aging subjects. Yet, contrary to this welfare-oriented "pastoral care" understanding, the reality of many nursing homes is quite different. This contrary viewpoint can be seen in that nursing homes often operate as speculative financial instruments or commodities in the corporatized health care market. According to Ettlinger, they were the first major institution to capitalize on an aging society, and they remain a forerunner in the ever-escalating privatization of U.S. health care.[105] In 2014, the Centers for Disease Control and Prevention (CDC) reported that 69.8 percent of nursing homes were for-profit, making them key "vehicles of investment."[106] Moreover, large firms outside of health care own many of these for-profit nursing homes, which became attractive precisely because they are so profitable.

Factors that led to the corporatization of nursing homes and their profitability are numerous. In the 1950s, the federal government established Federal Housing Authority mortgages that paid 90 percent of project costs for the construction of new nursing homes; by the 1960s, this resulted in a building boom in nursing home construction, exceeding the actual need among the elderly. This building investment operated essentially as a form of speculative real estate, with nursing home chains replacing smaller establishments and the sale of stock in these nursing home chains becoming a source of capital for the parent company. Of note is that these chains use complicated corporate structures that shield owners from lawsuits that might arise due to neglect or violations of legally imposed requirements for nursing home operation and care delivery.[107] A second core factor in the growing corporatization was the 1965 introduction of Medicare and Medicaid funding for short-term and long-term nursing home care, as previously noted. Per this funding, the federal government would cover the mortgage interest for nursing home facilities, enabling firms to use the initial mortgage on a property to finance the purchase of others in an operation known as pyramiding. This now-common occurrence—of multiple properties being owned by chain organizations—further obscures responsibility for substandard care and abuse.[108] Adding to the Medicare and Medicaid funding and assistance programs, the 1987 introduction of the Prospective Payment System (specifically DRG) incentivized fast hospital discharge to nursing homes for short-term stays, which in turn increased demand and contributed to the boom in construction. Important to note also is that as of 2002, 70 percent of networked companies or chains that owned nursing homes channeled revenues to other firms, essentially laundering money through the nursing home to other parts of the organization. This has enabled owners to claim that the institution operated at a loss and thus needed heightened government subsidies.[109] Through these brief examples, it becomes evident that the corporatization of nursing homes—and the economic incentives at work—often eclipses what many see as their core function: to provide pastoral care and secure the lives of the elderly infirm.

More than simply being compromised through corporatization, however, nursing homes often *work against* the very "make live" principle of contemporary biopolitics by providing what we call *deadly care.* Care in nursing homes can be deadly in a conceptual sense, in that it can engender social death—relegating the ill elderly outside the boundaries of community. In a more tangible sense, however, care can also be deadly when it curtails life—when it threatens life's continuance or when, in extreme cases, it results in premature death itself.

Revenue raising imperatives and cost-cutting rationalities of for-profit nursing homes (which, recall, are the majority) can be particularly detrimental to care—and, in many reported cases, deadly. Driven by the need to minimize costs of care and maximize profits, these institutions typically prefer short-term-stay residents because Medicare provides 84 percent more funding for these residents over Medicaid residents, who are longer-term, poor elderly individuals, often from underserved communities of color. Thus, many nursing homes move away from—and effectively abandon—longer-term end-of-life care for the elderly with extensive medical needs.[110] In some instances, nursing homes have also been known to exaggerate the therapy needs of short-term patients to acquire additional Medicare payments. The California-based chain Ensign Group had to pay $48 million in 2013 to settle such charges.[111] To attract these higher-funded patients, there is increasing investment in luxury facilities—such as the short-term-care wing of the Medford Multicare Center for Living on Long Island (known as the Lux at Medford); these facilities frequently include putting greens, "decadent hot baths," indoor parking, and other high-end rehabilitation amenities.[112] At the same time, however, minimizing the operational costs of facility operations is a key focus, resulting in cost cutting on meals and staff. This, in turn, leads to inflating the number of lower-paid nurse practitioners and aides, decreasing the number of on-site registered nurses, and often having no doctors on staff. What occurs, then, is a "chandelier effect," where the glitz of marketing promises does not match the actual quality of care—which is severely scaled back.

Moreover, *the delivery of care actually produces harm* under these conditions of extreme revenue raising and cost cutting. For example, a Department of Health and Human Services 2014 report found that 22 percent of Medicare patients who were residents of a nursing home for fewer than thirty-five days experienced harm from medical care while in such facilities. A further 11 percent suffered temporary injury.[113] Phillip C. Aka, Lucinda M. Deason, and Augustine Hammond speculate that such harm occurs in part because "nursing homes reaped lucrative profits as observable declines occurred in the care that they rendered to residents."[114] Furthermore, as more companies build nursing homes solely for short-term patients, many have been found to lack the capacity to deal with the specific and often acute medical needs of patients released from hospitals.[115]

Another way that care can be deadly in nursing homes results in part from the proceduralism involved in care delivery that addresses the biological body rather than a person with complex needs. Within these facilities, residents become a series of biological events that need to be monitored and accounted for under the medicalized gaze. Nursing home care primarily focuses on physical limitations and addressing incapacities rather than attending to the needs of the whole person, due in part to the medicalization of care but also to the documentation required of nursing homes by the government for them to continue to receive funding. Ettlinger describes the latter as "a maze of regulations that nurses and nurses' aides must navigate, resulting in a regime of practices of continually filling out forms."[116] Such documentation—for example, defecation books that are used to monitor and record the bowel movements of every patient—results in an endless bureaucracy of auditing, which in turn leads to decreased care. Care, which we might take to include conversation, attention—the minutiae of slow, careful assistance—is a liability to "efficiency" in this context, because it does not count toward government reimbursement. Thus, "in this light, abuse derives from actually following the rules."[117]

Several checks on the decline of care in nursing homes have been put in place to avoid harm being done to residents. The Nursing Home Reform Act of 1987 (at its inception) vested the Secretary of Health and Human Services with broad powers to address and enforce various standards of care, health, safety, and welfare/rights related to nursing homes and their residents in three main areas: care quality, inspection of facilities, and enforcement of newly introduced sanctions and fines for repeated violations. The Obama administration moved toward even tighter regulation of the health care system, which directly impacted nursing home care, though many of these measures are being wound back under the Trump administration.[118] Furthermore, hospitals now pay penalties if too many patients are readmitted, meaning that many are reticent to send discharged patients to nursing homes with poor records. Inadequate enforcement of these checks, however, is widely noted. A 2008 federal report, for instance, found that deficiencies (violations of a specific requirement for nursing home care) were missed at a rate of greater than 40 percent in all but five states, highlighting the ubiquity of deadly care.[119] The U.S. Government Accountability Report of 2015 found that deficiencies per nursing home surveyed had declined. At the same time, however, the report made clear that the average number of consumer complaints had actually risen, suggesting a discrepancy between clinical quality measures and patient and family experience—of ongoing deadly care.[120]

Hospice care is also ostensibly concerned with securing life: the goal is not primarily to make individuals live more but to achieve quality of life in the face of approaching death. This form of care is focused on optimizing *remaining* life—making the most of the time left, making this time as relatively pain-free as possible, and shepherding individuals toward death. In the United States, the hospice movement emerged in the mid-1970s, and by 1982, Congress had initiated a hospice benefit under the Tax Equity and Fiscal Responsibility Act, enabling hospice care to be included in the Medicare program. Core services of hospice include nursing care, personal assistance with ADLs, various forms of rehabilitation therapy, dietary counseling, psychosocial and spiritual counseling for both patient and family, volunteer services, respite care, provision of medical drugs and devices to alleviate pain and suffering from symptoms, and family bereavement services after the patient's death. Multidisciplinary care teams (nurses, social workers, pastoral counselors, and nursing assistants, among others) deliver this kind of care, operating under the management of either the patient's primary care physician or one affiliated with a hospice program. According to a National Hospice and Palliative Care Organization 2016 report on hospice patients from 2015, 44.4 percent died at home, 32.3 percent in a nursing facility, 15 percent in a hospice inpatient facility, and 7.6 percent in acute care within a hospital environment.[121] Importantly, hospice care repudiates the curative treatment model dominant in biomedicine to focus instead on palliative care. The reported benefits of this form of care are that it provides a more favorable dying experience compared with hospitalization, according to many family members;[122] delivers more personalized care plans than those available within a hospital environment;[123] and enables patients to live longer, with an average twenty-nine days reported over those who are hospitalized.[124]

Clearly hospice care appears as a positive and desirable form of care, one that would particularly aid the elderly infirm in their transition toward death. Yet, older individuals receiving such care can also be viewed as occupying the shadowlands, on the event horizon of life. In one sense, this can be seen in the scenario outlined by Julia Lawton, who notes that hospice care—particularly in a facility—is "progressively able only to cater for those patients who cannot be looked after within the community, because the community cannot accommodate them either practically or symbolically." She further argues that "it is not dying as such but, rather, certain kinds of deaths which are to be found within contemporary hospices."[125] The shadowlands in this context represent a sequestering of certain kinds of dying patients from the general populace, where the dying body is "dirty," ruptured, decaying—where the "unsightly" aspects of dying become visible.

The laudable goals of hospice care are further complicated by conditional and limited access. Medicare-enrolled individuals, for instance, are not able to begin hospice care until all curative treatments have been abandoned. Thus they must choose between what are positioned as polar pursuits—the elongation of life through treatment and those benefits that hospice provides. Limited access is seen in that only 1 percent of hospice services are free for those without insurance, and while 85.5 percent of patients access hospice care through Medicare, 76 percent of those patients are white, fewer than half the hospitals in rural areas have hospice programs, and less than 5 percent of those categorized as "urban poor" receive such care in their last six months of life. Furthermore, 11 million undocumented immigrants are legally barred from enrolling in any federally funded insurance program, meaning that they cannot access the end-of-life care offered by hospice services.[126]

Even if individuals can access hospice care, it is increasingly governed by financial logics that can be deadly for patients. For instance, between 2001 and 2008, the for-profit hospice industry grew 128 percent, while the nonprofit sector grew only 1 percent. As of 2008, 52 percent of hospice organizations were for profit, 35 percent were nonprofit, and 13 percent were government owned.[127] This for-profit sector only continued to expand, with the CDC reporting that as of 2014, 60.2 percent of hospice delivery programs or organizations were for profit.[128] Again, such for-profit companies are beholden to their investors, and the implicit profit-making imperatives at work often threaten to compete with patient and family care. Rather than securing the remaining life of patients, what is increasingly being secured is the financial gain of the for-profit industry. This profit pursuit can be seen along two primary avenues: first, hospice providers delimit the kinds of care available, and, particularly in a for-profit operation, they can withhold care as they try to stay within the set funding amounts that they receive through Medicare. For example, expensive diagnostic tests that could find sources of pain (and enable the alleviation of patient discomfort) are often denied by hospice corporations to improve their profit margins. The Medicare funding structure can also mean that hospice providers come to exaggerate the forms of care given to bill Medicare for higher reimbursements that are then channeled back into the company rather than toward patients. Second, patients themselves can be viewed as vehicles of extraction, as evident in various instances of hospice companies recruiting individuals for hospice care (while in hospital) to inflate the company's Medicare billings. In late 2017, for example, Chemed Corp. and Vitas Hospice Services agreed to pay $75 million to resolve charges relating to their practice of both billing for ineligible patients and reporting to Medicare for inflated levels of care.[129] Chemed—the largest provider of hospice services in the United States (operating forty-six facilities across fifteen states and the District of Columbia)—reportedly sent employees to nursing homes under the instruction to recruit patients and then rewarded those employees with bonuses for the additional number of patients they brought in for hospice care. Another hospice provider "was indicted for allegedly paying nursing home operators $10 per day to assist in patient recruitment efforts and paying physicians $89 a month to certify patients as hospice eligible without examining the patient or reviewing medical records."[130] In such cases, profiteering eclipses care, and the original philosophy and ethics behind hospice are abandoned—along with the patients.

Ultimately, these arenas where the dependent elderly are meant to receive assistance in securing life, or what life remains, are overshadowed by neoliberal biopolitical logics that render a social problem (infirmity in old age) as an economic opportunity. Both nursing homes and hospice can be seen to present possibilities for corporate welfare over social welfare, wherein the elderly infirm actually become vehicles for financial extraction. These arenas also overshadow care—their ostensible purpose. The proceduralism and cost accounting that are central to neoliberalism and the daily operations of these spaces actually work against the affirmation to secure by engendering deadly forms of care.

Counterconducts of Aging

The field of "critical gerontology" has raised important criticisms of the ways normative ideas about "successful aging" and anti-aging exacerbate social injustices and may even undermine aspects of our humanity.[131] This chapter has sought to contribute to such discussions of justice and aging by foregrounding how processes that attempt to elongate and secure life can produce various forms of insecure senior citizenship and intensify inequalities in old age—even leading to harmful practices in eldercare and death. Although we have not provided an exhaustive account of U.S. biocultures of aging, we have examined several key aspects of the governmentality of aging, from the aging body and self to the aging population, from third age promotional rhetoric to the shadowlands of fourth age abandonment. Third age discourse and health metrics repudiate impairment and dependency and marginalize disabled individuals as nonproductive and thus "dysfunctional." Affirming functional aging and independent seniors may justify a biopolitics of disposability of aging subjects who do not, or who are unable to, access technical aids or biomedical life extensions that maintain self-sufficiency and productivity—and who cannot align themselves with an escalating utilitarian health economics. The governance of dying bodies and bodies in decline in nursing homes and hospices, in particular, exposes variable gaps between "human" and "citizen": individual bodies undergoing care in deep age, hovering between life and death, remain invested with rights but simultaneously risk exploitation and neglect. Moreover, citizen status stratifies the senior population and is itself insecure and stratified. Many elder bodies—poor seniors, elders of color, elderly women, immigrant seniors, LGBTQ elders, and so forth—fall into what Matthew Sparke calls "biological subcitizenship" in relation to national and global health regimes, wherein power relations and different mechanisms of exclusion, conditioning, and extraction shape aging. Aging is thus biological *and* a process of embodying differential degrees of health rights disenfranchisement and political–economic subordination.[132]

Our analysis focused on the deathly effects of affirming life in the face of aging and the deathly conditions that some people experience within the U.S. security apparatus against aging. However, we want to make clear that the compression of morbidity and alleviation of the pain of decline and dying are not "bad": mitigating aging is linked to the biomedical ethical imperative to reduce suffering.[133] Nor do we draw a line on the extent to which life-extending medical procedures should be used in late life or whether preempting aging, disease, and death via strategies of detection and successful aging results in more harm than good. Instead, our goal has been to locate openings for critical reflection on the governance of aging, old age, and decline. A primary concern is the encroaching forms of "morbid life" and subjection to deadly forms of care and predatory financial exploitation that old people—among the most vulnerable segments of the population—may now experience in the very institutions where processes of aging and dying are addressed and largely sequestered, that is, hospitals, nursing homes, and hospices. Policies that define aging as a security problem and actively influence these institutions often draw on economic accounting metrics and quantitative techniques of population management that position the elderly as with no future and whose years of life are valued less (for compromising economic productivity potential), unless capacitated through biomedical or technical interventions that "overcome" decline and disability. The dominant emphasis of third age discourse on "aging well"—to help people live more through activity regimes and other individualized disciplinary pursuits of volunteering, lifelong learning, and so on—essentially positions the degenerative capacity and dependency of old age as unacceptable. If to age well is to *not* have trouble, suffering, or cares—to not be vulnerable or subject to bodily precarity—then, as this chapter has argued, efforts to age well are value-laden and carry potentially negative effects, perhaps best exemplified by the alarming prevalence of militant rhetoric exhorting individuals to "combat aging."[134] In late liberal conditions, the maintenance of functional aging and healthy living has become part of the life work of each active citizen, with other modes of aging disregarded and even pathologized.[135]

What are our obligations across generations?[136] In response to these security problematics of aging, how might an "emancipatory gerontology" work against the grain, counteracting the prizing of individualism and self-responsibilization of risk in favor of dependency, interrelatedness, and recognition of shared vulnerability? What practices, ethics, and social relations of aging demonstrate care and love for the oldest generations outside frameworks of economic metrics, medical treatments, consumerism, and offloading the elderly to the corporate shadows? What models of empathy and connectivity would revalue aging as integral to society and the lifeworld of the population, particularly where age functions as a mutable political and social threshold "between surplus and waste, obsolescence and renewal?"[137] How might recognizing—rather than repudiating—differential but mutually shared vulnerability across the life-span reposition the elderly as positive contributors and mentors who can reveal something invaluable about life, its contingencies, and adaptation—including how to live in a dying body and how to secure a "good death" as a social rather than merely individual project?

A promising pedagogical innovation that may inspire an ethics of empathy toward the everyday experience of living with an aging body is AgeLab's suit AGNES—the "Age Gain Now Empathy System." Donning the suit equips the wearer with the prosthetic limitations of a seventy-year-old body.[138] A short video demonstration on the AgeLab website explains, "This suit was designed to provide insight into the physical effects of aging.... Put on this suit and you feel increased fatigue, reduced flexibility in joints and muscles, spinal compression, and difficulty with vision and balance."[139] The idea is that the suit will allow designers, planners, product developers, architects, packaging engineers, and so on, to experience the challenges associated with aging for themselves; it is a method for investigating how a product, service, and/or environment is navigated and used by an older adult. AGNES gestures toward a design culture and, more broadly, popular culture that teaches empathy through creative prosthesis applications,

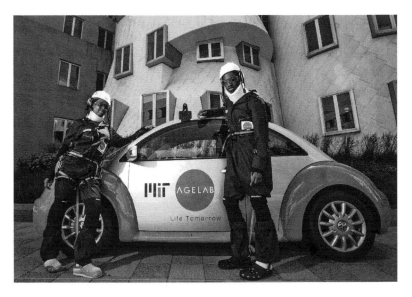

Figure 12. AgeLab's AGNES suit. Photograph courtesy of MIT AgeLab.

experimenting with disability aesthetics to reposition interdependency and rethink agency and autonomy within social relations. AGNES represents one effort to design things through assisting and exploring—rather than denying or "solving"—a future that is accessible and engaging to the elderly and bodies with special mobility and motor function requirements.

Activism strategies around aging in the policy arena build on the U.S. civil rights movement by establishing multigenerational support for "elder councils" and other institutions that would hold old age in esteem and by advocating economic and health justice for people of all ages. The Gray Panthers, for example, have established a series of intergenerational advocacy networks across the United States that confront ageism and social justice issues, including challenging ageist laws, such as a mandatory retirement age; Medicare and Social Security preservation; multigenerational cohousing; the fair treatment of people in nursing homes; and racism in the aging policy-making arena.[140] Since its establishment in 1970 and early admiration for the militancy of the Black Panthers, the Gray Panthers continue to be at the forefront of provocative demands that reject the docile acceptance of how social relations and institutions are organized to abandon, exploit, or generally repudiate the elderly and the laborers who care for the vulnerable elderly.[141] The Diverse Elders Coalition, formed in 2010, advocates for policies and programs that improve aging for the diverse communities that compose the U.S. population, targeting economic insecurity among older adults of color and LGBTQ elders in particular.[142] The coalition has directed campaigns to increase support for family caregivers who provide unpaid care labor so that family members, friends, and neighbors can age with health and dignity: for example, a dependent care credit that individuals who spend part of their working years caring for elderly family members can apply toward their Social Security earnings.[143] The organization also seeks to close competency gaps that inhibit paid caregivers from providing the best care to diverse elders and to reform the U.S. immigration system by supplying more employment visas to domestic care workers as a high-needs sector and by creating more inclusive pathways to citizenship for this critical labor sector.[144] These policy-directed efforts challenge U.S. biocultures of aging by focusing on the structural conditions of caregiving and by rejecting a limited clinical biomedical model of health and aging for an explicitly political framework of social justice.

Experiments with elderly commons, cohousing networks, and time-banking eschew corporate nursing homes and isolated smart homes for alternative social and intergenerational arrangements of space and time. Resident-created retirement solutions take various forms, from shared homes to communes, multigenerational housing to neighborhoods of people who watch out for each other and take on shared responsibility for meals, errands, and care. The national Village to Village movement—"a peer-to-peer grassroots network run by volunteers and paid staff to coordinate services such as transportation, home repairs, shopping trips, and social opportunities among seniors who live independently in their own homes"—reportedly reached more than 150 villages operating across the United States, with more than a hundred in development as of 2015.[145] "Intentional communities"—an umbrella term for living situations organized around a common vision or value structure—also known as "cohousing," conceptually migrated to the United States in the 1980s after originating in Denmark decades earlier.[146] While earlier models have been artist collectives and religious or self-help communes, cohousing is a growing practice of increasing interest to young and old alike.[147] Cohousing, by design, basically entails *aging in community*—a social agreement of mutual aid and care, whereby people willingly agree to live in a way that depends on others and supports others. The popularity of cohousing reveals that the trend

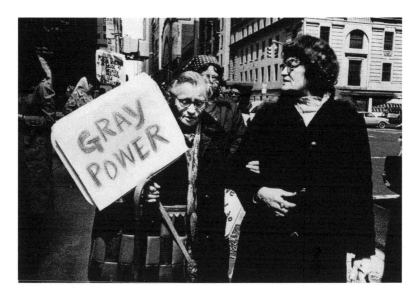

Figure 13. Gray Panthers demonstrate for better living conditions, 1975. Photograph by Bettye Lane. Schlesinger Library, Radcliffe Institute, Harvard University.

of people seeking to age in place, to avoid institutionalization and remain in a home environment for as long as possible, does not necessarily mean an unquestioned acceptance of the risks and costs of this kind of independence. For many rising seniors, robo-equipped homes and the mental health deterioration caused by isolated and segregated "elderly islands" are not acceptable trade-offs for independence.[148] Moreover, the lofty expenses of safety modifications that make individual homes accessible and of nursing care to each person's home make cohousing and cost sharing desirable. Thus "home share can provide companionship, save costs, and enhance security—as a cost-effective alternative to isolated home care."[149]

The Cohousing Association of the United States—which reported more than 150 cohousing member communities in 2015, stretching from Fairbanks, Alaska, to Atlanta, Georgia—inaugurated an Aging in Cohousing initiative in 2017 to support the creation of age-friendly cohousing communities and physical and social environments across the United States, where people can "flourish as they get older."[150] A roommate-linking service that references a mid-1980s-era TV sitcom about senior women sharing housing—the Golden Girls Roommate Network—remains an active resource for adults, especially women, to locate housemates and arrange co-habitation.[151] Among the poorest segment of the population—often without retirement funds and unable to cover at-home care because they spent their lives caring for families—many women are creating their own retirement communities and practicing exclusively female, self-governing cohousing.[152] For example, the Baba Yaga House—first developed in a Parisian suburb in 2012—incorporated more than twenty women ages sixty-six to eighty-nine, with one-third of them living on the poverty line—into an apartment building where each performed chores and pooled resources for medical staff.[153] Named after a supernatural being in Slavic folklore who offers advice to younger women, the Baba Yaga House has traveled to North America, specifically Toronto, among women who want to live independently and cooperatively into old age within a community.[154] With core principles of mutual care, shared governance, feminism and social justice, interdependence, community engagement, and environmental responsibility, the women's cohousing project—in its original and subsequent iterations—exercises an intergenerational commitment through hosting open university courses and other events.[155]

Intergenerational housing and cooperatives can foster empathy for the declining body and secure social responsibility for the oldest population. There are communes, such as the Fellowship Community near Manhattan, that serve as alternatives to assisted living homes and hospices, where palliative care is undertaken by the community.[156] Many U.S. families increasingly live with multiple generations under one roof, often to provide family-based senior care and cut down on costs; while most of these families live in ordinary houses, the home-building industry is responding quickly to the shifting demand by creating homes and metro-oriented developments geared toward multigenerational living.[157] Beyond family or fellowship cohousing, intergenerational shared services and spaces can promote the dignity of seniors and mobilize co-mentoring and social interdependence. Timebanking, for example, values the time of senior participants as much as anyone else, encouraging reciprocity through helping and trading aid through a social network that treats everyone as an asset.[158] Timebanks are a community of people who have agreed to trade each other their services, usually based on time as the currency (i.e., one hour of a computer specialist equals one hour of a domestic worker).[159] One manifestation of timebanking is combining elderly care centers with preschools. For instance, the Intergenerational Learning Centre in West Seattle administers a preschool within a senior center that is home to more than four hundred elderly residents; the very young and old share lunches and a curriculum in music, dancing, art, and storytelling.[160] Another possibility would be inviting young people to assist in nursing homes and elderly communities as a means to bank time—and thus earn credits—toward their own retirement, in the process broadening their perspectives on life, death, and the different ways that people navigate old age and its associated physical changes.[161] In general, projects that locate university students and/or young families in nursing homes and cross-generational co-ops can both reduce living costs and improve care through timebanking.[162] Generations United, an organization that supports intergenerational projects, lists numerous other cohabitation options: community centers with programs for multiple generations, adult day care and child care programs housed in the same facility, programs for disadvantaged youth run through a nursing home. Central to its mission is overcoming barriers that stem from the way U.S. funding streams and zoning or other regulatory requirements assume that segregating generations is socially desirable and correct protocol.[163]

Finally, adoption offers a way to revalue the elderly. Many faith-based groups run "adopt-a-grandparent" and "adopt-a-senior" programs, and some high schools and universities offer school credit to youth who visit nursing homes and assisted living facilities and pair up with senior residents to spend time with them.[164] The more progressive programs encourage co-mentoring and co-learning experiences that are mutually beneficial to both partners, emphasizing the importance of social bonds and sorting out what matters in life and in facing death.[165] Michel Foucault advocated for an even more radical right of adult adoption. Speaking in the context of rights claims about sexuality, Foucault argued that rights are not simply statements of universal truths but rather are performative practices that can "contest conventional ways of thinking about who we are, whom we should love, and how we should use our bodies . . . [and question] the dominant norms of relationships and practices of care."[166] As Ben Golder explains, Foucault bitingly criticizes the tenets of liberal individualism upon which rights politics are said to rest, as well as the unimaginative claim that rights politics are merely about limiting the power of the state to control the lives of individuals; instead, rights claims can challenge the ways that we live as much as domesticate them.[167] Thus, claiming the right to adult adoption— and using the language of rights—might perform critical "counterconduct" that challenges conceptions of marriage and families and other structures of life that are often taken for granted as inevitable.[168] The future of aging and the elderly involves nothing less than imagining and putting into practice alternative relations of care and obligation among people—beyond marriage and family and what may even count as normal and natural relationships.[169] Karen Zivi elaborates on the challenge and potential reward: "the right to adult adoption would question these accepted relationships while expanding the possibilities for living together and caring for others. It would bring into existence a new way of understanding intimate relations of care and dependency, allowing us to 'escape as much as possible from the type of relations that society proposes for us and try to create . . . new relational possibilities.'"[170] Together, these alternative biocultures of aging reimagine what it means to secure life in old age, suggesting an expansive range of possibilities that attend to, play with, and revere vulnerability and relationality.

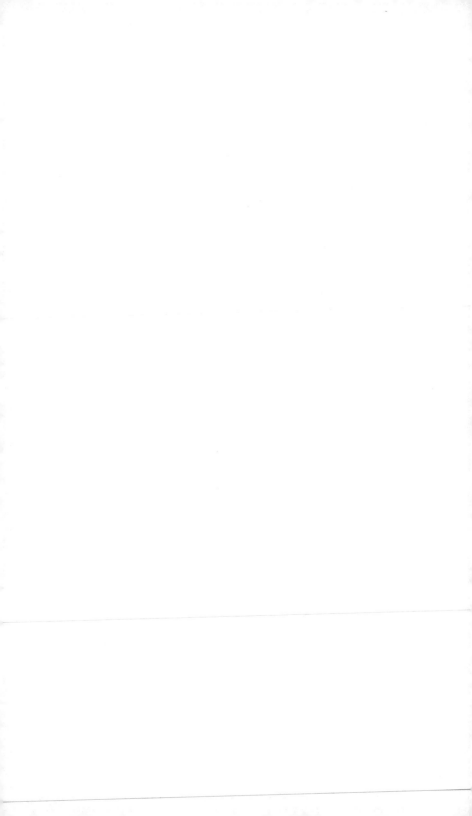

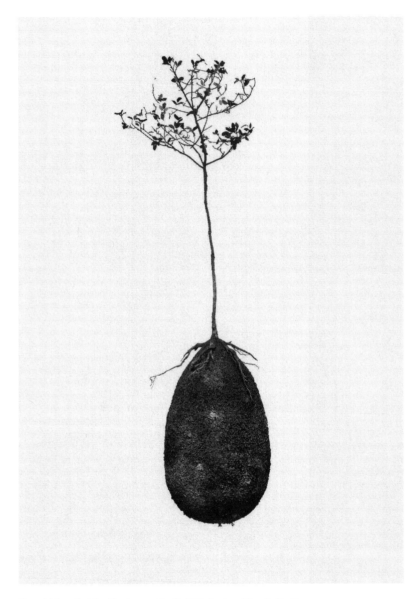

Figure 14. Green burial pod/environmental coffin, 2012. Courtesy of Capsula Mundi.

5

Green

Death

*As the rhetoric of "green" choice surrounds us, nothing will be spared, not
even death.*

—Suzanne Kelly, "Dead Bodies That Matter"

*The bodies of black people, convicts, women, the insane and the poor
have been differentially treated, reminding us of the need constantly to
situate reflections on our shared humanity in contexts of conquest and
dispossession—as much of the corpse as of living subjects.*

—Deborah Posel and Pamila Gupta, "The Life of the Corpse"

This book has examined *life-making practices* that affirm life and intimately
govern through a regulatory politics of affirmation. People are called on to
participate in such life-making as if it is unquestionably good, rather than
an intensification of stratified living or subjection of bodies to new risks.
The previous chapters explored how life-making simultaneously creates
deathly conditions and obscures death. In a politics that is focused on
affirming life, death is invisibilized. But we can also see that in death, the
body enters regulatory processes of affirmation, namely, a material afterlife
that is subject to power relations. Increased proceduralization of dying and
the event of death within U.S. biomedicine undoubtedly demonstrates an
"assemblage of techniques of power designed to reproduce and discipline
human populations"—including dead populations.[1] Even more so, the disposal and commemoration of human remains reveal that death does not
lie beyond the reach of power: bodies *remain* after death, and a variety of
cultural practices, technologies, and administrative interventions aim to
resolve this "remaining."[2] Considering the eventful fate of dead bodies oc-
casions a critical juncture in which to explore both the biopolitical management of material remains and the disciplining of the very materiality of the
dead body. The governance of the dead points to some of the ways that the

dead body has been understood—that is, the range of practices that administer and discipline the corpse in U.S. society—as an economic input in the funeral industry, material waste to be eliminated, a resource for the living and a form of property, a quasi-subject to be granted respect and privacy, and an active medium of connection between the living and deceased.[3] This chapter focuses on the changing administration of human remains that emphasizes material–biological extraction and ecological legacy.[4] We argue that such death practices show how—*even in death*—life (of some people or in some form) is affirmed *as afterlife* unevenly and with contradictory benefits. Put another way, our claim here is that the biomedical commitment to affirming life extends into the administration of death and the disciplining of the dead body. Thus, even when released from biomedicine's grasp, life is affirmed—as afterlife. This affirmation of life (in death) is, however, still regulatory; it still stratifies populations; and it still disavows the recognition of certain deaths and lives lived.

The chapter investigates biocultures of afterlife that, we argue, are increasingly subjected to the *affirmation to "green" death and the dead body.* Environmental sustainability concerns are reconfiguring American death care: handling the dead body has expanded into a vibrant field of disposal and commemoration activities that address issues of sustainability, toxicity, waste, land scarcity, and global warming, in addition to legacy and memorialization. The affirmation to "green" at the final frontier of life seeks to make death sustainable through intensified *bioremediation* of the dead body: the reuse and reprocessing of dead bodies/parts and the conversion of afterlife to forms of value beyond death.[5] We survey bioremediation practices that affirm the afterlife of the corpse as an opportunity to commemorate sustainability as personal legacy, generate new markets and efficiencies, and secure particular environmental legacies and relations between the living and the dead. We delineate two ways that bioremediation expands the governance of dead bodies/parts and their material possibilities for biovalue. First, some disposal efforts encourage an economy of body/parts beyond death and a utilitarian ethic of efficiency—"no remains." Accordingly, the afterlife is not "the end" but a renewable material resource and opportunity to economize the body in death and put the dead body to work. Here greening the afterlife of the corpse refers to ecological and commercial imperatives that advocate reusing the dead body and reintegrating the waste generated through cremation technologies into alternative energy infrastructure—specifically, reprocessing crematorium heat waste, recycling orthopedic implants, and gifting corporeal value through whole-body or organ donation. Second, we observe a range of practices that reimagine death as an opportunity for personal legacy and redeem the body's decomposition as natural/as part of the natural world. Bioremediation in this case conceptually recuperates death into life so that death is not wasted. From green burial practices to the integration of cremation ashes or human DNA in new corporeal–memorial life-forms, such as "eternal reefs" and "transgenic tombstones," the corpse serves as a material input for nature and a vehicle for legacy—what we refer to as *biopresence*.[6] The material vitality of the body "lives on" through customized postmortem commemoration that validates the value of a life through claims of environmental benefits.

How bodies affect our environments today will impact people and land-scapes in years to come. As indicated by the second opening quote to this chapter, U.S. governance of the dead has historically entailed the differential treatment of bodies *after* life: some dead bodies are privately preserved and remembered; others have been stolen and displayed or studied. In this context, the greening of death and affirmation of the dead body's afterlife through bioremediation practices have social, political, and environmental consequences, including potentially advancing the biopolitics of dispos-ability and erasure of bodies subject to "bad deaths."[7] This chapter therefore considers some of the paradoxes and potential costs of greening the dead in order to galvanize awareness of social justice issues that operate across the living and the dead—in other words, to promote "death equity" appraisals at the intersections of environmental justice and what Clare Madge calls "relational mortality."[8] Bioremediation laudably demonstrates an ethical and/or economic commitment to affirming the greening of the body's af-terlife. Yet this activity also risks legitimating the status quo characterized by excessive consumption, orchestrating efficiencies for a predatory death industry, and obscuring a long history of biopiracy and experimentation on racial minorities. While greening the disposal of one's own body—to leave a sustainable or green legacy—is viewed as a gift to nature, the underside of this operation is further entrenchment of social position in life and an intensified legacy of violent human–nonhuman and person–thing social divisions in the landscape.

The point of our speculative venture into the arena of the afterlife in this final chapter is not to totalize or wholesale criticize efforts to make death more sustainable or affirm it as natural. Many green death projects are commendable, creative, and necessary interventions in a pervasively death-averse culture. Our aim, however, is to reflect on these bioreme-diation efforts through the lens of what Michel Foucault referred to as "caesuras" within biopolitics that *make some lives not matter in life—or, we argue, in afterlife*.[9] While he was referring to racism—and we remain interested in the idea of the "racial cut" that stratifies the population in death just as in life—our broader interest is to consider how affirming the afterlife ostensibly enhances inequalities of the living and buttresses a politics of expungement that rules out the possibility of a "good death" for certain individuals and communities. In response to the potential so-cial hazards presented by "sustainable death" practices, particularly ra-cialized and class-based exclusions, we ask: what possibilities exist for an environmental ethics of human remains that contributes to—rather than obscures—environmental justice and civil rights projects? We conclude by querying how conduct for the dead might advance social justice through a material politics of human remains.

U.S. Biocultures of Death Care: A Brief Environmental History

A brief environmental history of U.S. death care contextualizes concerns today about the negative impacts of the standard American way of death, that is, earth burial of embalmed bodies and the increasingly popular flame-based cremation. The affirmation to green death both challenges and pres-ents tremendous opportunity for the well-entrenched death industry, sig-naling significant reforms in the governance of the dead. Essentially, dead human bodies experience a material afterlife. This afterlife is organized and governed by death work and funerary practices, most notably a national (now transnational) funeral industry focused on the perishable body.[10] Death care expertise in the United States historically removed deathly ritu-als and the dead body from everyday home life to medical institutions and a formalized funeral profession.[11] Legitimated by the rise of mortuary sci-ence, professional death work would come to offer specialized services that handled disposal of the dead, mitigated perceived health concerns, and expanded commemoration through time and space with a growing market of memorial products and services.

The cultural–economic rise of this death care industry is often attributed to the "post-bellum reconstruction of America (1865–1880) and the rising power of corporations in constructing the hegemony of consumption."[12] Since the American Civil War, embalming of the corpse has anchored the configuration of the American funeral industry, with emphasis on improving the material aesthetics, "shelf life," and geographical range of dead bodies as chemically preserved fleshy artifacts conferred with postmortem subjectivity.[13] The Civil War generated thousands of dead bodies and resulted in the material problem of how to return them home.[14] In response, embalming expedited technological domination over space and time, to forestall decay and enable corpses to travel and continue to meaningfully reference the deceased. A professional–managerial class of funeral directors helped to formalize the new market and supply chain for death services. The progressively commodified funeral process was further bolstered by an increase in wealth among a middle class that could pay for death care. Central to the industry, embalming and refrigeration enabled the transportation of the dead body, while innovations from the telegraph to coffin catalogs connected the living to the dead through an array of funerary rituals and product options.

As the role of the funerary professional came to be associated with science and the medical establishment, techno-funerary practices affected new corpse geographies and "deathscapes" in relation to the American landscape.[15] American cultural distance from death over the course of the twentieth century spurred the routine movement of the dead from hospital bed to funeral home to memorial park. Control and containment of the corpse served the dual purpose of removing and intervening in the unruly nature of decomposition to eradicate the (real or perceived) health hazards of dead bodies and of converting the corpse into a mobile "commodity" that could aggregate myriad other commemorative commodities (elaborate coffins, tombstones, urns, etc.). Even cremation, which was seldom used in comparison with traditional burial in the United States, was initially heralded in the rhetoric of sanitation. Attendant to the professionalized handling of the corpse, the cemetery transitioned from a largely local communal sacred space—where the living and the dead were separated but symbolically joined through memorial rites—to a distant, private, secular, and commercialized landscape. Memorial parks, in particular, functioned to sequester and sanitize the dead body within a highly ordered environment and (industrially) maintained pastoral scenery outside of middle-class urban living; its ornamental nature "was viewed as a moral virtue destined to make city life less harsh."[16] Removed from the home and local graveyard, the memorial park offered a final resting place for dead bodies and their visitors—usually in the form of family-grouped individual plots of land or memorial niches purchased in a columbarium or community mausoleum for "cremains." The aesthetics and regulations of the landscape were used to market and manage the cemetery as well as to secure an attractive and sacred space for funerary practice, thereby distancing the morbid connotations of the cemetery.[17] In short, American burial practices and deathscapes have emphasized containment of the dead body and preservation of static environments for the dead removed from everyday life.[18]

The resources required for this way of death draw attention to its environmental impact: Americans annually bury more than 30 million board feet of hardwood (caskets), more than one hundred thousand tons of steel, copper, and bronze (caskets and vaults), more than eight hundred thousand gallons of embalming fluid, and 1.6 million tons of reinforced concrete.[19] Caskets and vaults may contaminate soil and groundwater by leaching preservatives, sealants, and metals. Furthermore, cemeteries are typically beautified with turf and kept verdant via regular applications of pesticides and fertilizers.[20] Not only can cemeteries be toxic, particularly for workers, but the spread of embalming fluid and other inert chemicals throughout the gravesite environment also inhibits human death from contributing to the landscape through decay. That is, the sanitized corpse is placed outside of the decomposition that it could undergo in the soil due to the way funerary technologies destroy important microbes and ward off insects necessary for the breakdown of the body.[21] A sustainable death movement today, in part, arose to reverse the distancing of the corpse and repudiation of its decay and to reimagine deathly ritual and legacy in environmentally friendly forms.

One such reimagining has been cremation, which Americans have increasingly preferred to burial. Between 1960 and 2010, U.S. cremation rates increased from 3.56 to 40.6 percent: the rate reached 45.4 percent in 2013 and is projected to surpass burial by almost three times by 2030.[22] Many Americans favor cremation for its efficiency and reduced environmental impact; it is often touted as the "clean" alternative to burial's perceived environmental and consumer rights threats, such as expensive maintenance of scarce burial grounds, the desire to save land, or the neo-Malthusian view that there are too many humans (alive or dead).[23] Yet several studies have shown the toxic effects of crematoria, namely, elevated mercury levels in crematory worker hair and the soils surrounding the buildings near crematoria.[24] Not only does the incineration process use massive amounts of nonrenewable energy sources to maintain the furnace but it also generates carbon dioxide and numerous noxious gases and carcinogens.[25] Contaminants—embalming fluid (usually a mix of formaldehyde, methanol, and ethanol); radioactive isotopes from cancer treatments; vaporized mercury emissions from dental fillings; silicone from breast implants; or harmful accumulations of zinc, copper, or iron—eventually make their way into the atmosphere. Wasting of heat/energy through a polluting incineration process has warranted environmental opposition in recent decades and catalyzed efforts to make cremation more efficient and clean-burning.

In response to death care services and technologies deemed to be toxic, inefficient, wasteful, excessive, deleterious to natural/ecological processes, and/or exploitative, a wide spectrum of green death practices—that intersect with and reflect broader social and economic pursuits of "sustainability" in late capitalism—now seek to expend fewer resources and reduce the environmental and economic burden of death's administration.[26] As the rest of this chapter will explore, the greening of death demonstrates changing biopolitical governance of dead bodies as material resources to be converted to other uses as well as shifting attitudes toward the nature of the human body and death—their role and place in society—and new norms of commemoration and conduct for the dead.

Sustainable Death: Bioremediation of the Dead Body

If traditionally the governing of death emphasized containment of the dead body, we now see practices that remediate the material afterlife—that convert and exploit dead bodies.[27] Bioremediation of the dead body and body parts reorganizes the body after death—conceptually and materially—for purposes that range from alternative energy infrastructure projects that operate at the biopolitical level, to new memorial life-forms that operate more at the level of individual bodies. We observe two overlapping trends—what we call "no remains" and "biopresence"—that simultaneously show the material afterlife of the corpse: as new forms of biovalue harnessed at the scale of the population and as ways to discipline and *make productive* the dead body beyond the life of a subject—beyond death. With this conceptual schema, we wish to underscore the material processes and power relations that govern the body's afterlife—the material nature of dead human bodies and our relations with the material remains of the dead. In the first case, the afterlife presents an opportunity to economize the body in death and put the dead body to work in new ways as a material resource.

To "green" death here entails new markets and efficiencies as the source of biovalue. We examine a few examples of the bioremediation of the corpse that can be seen to affirm life in the broader social arena, such as orthopedic implant recycling and heat-waste reprocessing at crematoria. The second case briefly explores death practices that redefine the corpse as a material contribution to nature and vehicle for personal legacy. These efforts seek to conceptually recuperate death-in-life so that death is not wasted—nor lays waste to nature. From green burial to memorial trees, we examine efforts to reimagine honoring the dead through interactions with land/nature and new technologies that implant postmortem human presence. In short, the governance of death now affirms a material afterlife of efficiency, utility, adaptation, and exploitation of dead bodies for entrepreneurial purposes and/or personal legacy.[28]

No Remains

The usefulness of dead bodies and their constituent parts spans a long history, including the supply of cadavers for medical schools, donations of bodies to science, and the circulation and regulation of organs for transplant. The intensification of this general trajectory can be seen in current repurposing efforts that strive to produce "no remains" by getting the most out of the body after death. A bio-economy of body parts beyond the life of the subject has expanded transnationally to service biotech enterprises and new cadaver-sourced bioproducts, such as "face transplants, cadaver collagen beauty treatments, genomics, stem cell research, organ harvesting"— challenging the definition and limits of the proper use of the corpse.[29] Motivations for these efforts interrelate economic and ethical imperatives: for some, it is about transforming the dead body into forms of biovalue via enhanced efficiencies within broader circuits of capital. As Catherine Waldby explains, biovalue is generated whenever the productivity of life/ living entities—in this case, dead bodies and their material afterlife—can be instrumentalized in ways that are useful to human projects.[30] There is also an ethical orientation at work that strives to recast death, advocating for the reprocessing of dead bodies and body parts. "No remains" thus covers a spectrum of activities that aim to convert the material afterlife of the corpse as waste into energy, infrastructure, or scientific or forensic gift.

Organ donation is an obvious starting point for considerations of the affirmation of the dead body and its corporeal value to the living.[31] More than 145 million people in the United States were registered as donors in

2018, to supply replacement parts for the bodies of the living.[32] Even though waitlisted patients exceed donors by nearly tenfold, more than eighty-five hundred deceased donors in 2014 enabled approximately twenty-four thousand organ transplants, along with nearly forty-eight thousand corneal transplants and more than 1 million tissue transplants.[33] The biosciences have also put the corpse to work in anatomical models and forensic evidence, asking people "to consider anatomical gifts as your last charitable act."[34] For example, the Anatomy Bequest Program of the renowned Mayo Clinic "accepts whole-body donations for the purposes of medical education, research and surgical training, and the development and testing of new surgical devices and techniques."[35] Another whole-body donation option supports the study of human decomposition at one of the country's taphonomic facilities ("body farms") to advance forensic science of human remains.[36] The leading outdoor laboratory of cadaver decay at the University of Tennessee boasts a predonor waiting list of nearly three thousand individuals from all fifty states and six different countries.[37]

Far outstripping forensics body donation numbers, cremation in the United States now figures prominently in a consumer-based ethics to reduce the material footprint of humans after death. Orthopedic recycling and waste-to-energy reprocessing at crematoria represent efforts to harness and redirect taken-for-granted or unacknowledged material waste streams, with complex motives spanning explicit for-profit gain and humanitarian charity. "No remains" in these scenarios means reducing the waste produced via the cremation process. Human bodies are becoming more industrial in life and afterlife—an ontological position that Donna Haraway referred to as the "cyborg."[38] Dead bodies contain metal joints, mercury dental fillings, surgical materials, silicone breast implants, pacemaker batteries, and numerous inorganic elements. Cremation presents an opportunity to collect, sort, and melt down valuable metal by-products that formerly operated in the body before death (from titanium hips to cobalt-chrome knees). After being subject to fifteen hundred to eighteen hundred degree Fahrenheit cremation temperatures, recovered metals are sold on the global manufacturing market, with proceeds returned to the crematorium or a selected charity.[39] For example, Detroit-based Implant Recycling LLC, owned by a fourth-generation family of metal recyclers, works with twelve hundred crematoria, providing bins, sending out a company delivery truck to pick them up for collection back in Detroit, and offering crematoria compensation for their time and effort.[40] Within the 65 percent of U.S. crematoria that now recycle medical prostheses, some companies emphasize obtaining consent from the deceased's family or representative and the ethical choice to recycle (even though it may take a for-profit form), while others advocate a strictly nonprofit approach of giving joint recycling proceeds to charity.[41]

This emphasis on efficiency and utility in what we might see as the biopolitical governance of afterlife in late liberalism has led to upgrades in cremation technology and infrastructure. For example, reprocessing the heat generated by cremation has revamped crematoria designs that remain largely based in the nineteenth century. Pragmatic efforts to comply with emission reduction requirements (mercury and dioxins) and generate alternative energy sources are pushing for revisions to cremation conveyance.[42] Europe and Asia lead the charge in making profitable use of excess heat that would otherwise be wasted, with new cremator technologies that convert waste heat from incineration into electricity.[43] A typical cremation generates between two hundred and four hundred kilowatts of waste heat that can be harnessed to warm cemetery roads and chapels or converted to chill freezers or air condition waiting rooms in crematoria.[44] The cremation division of Florida-based Matthews International is working on a U.S. application that would transform waste heat into electrical energy that can be put back on the grid.[45] The United States only recuperates about 12 percent of its heat, in part because trapped heat cannot travel far and the majority of the country's centralized power plants are further from urban centers than their European and Asian counterparts.[46] With U.S. cremation figures projected to reach 71 percent by 2030, crematoria present growth industry potential for transforming yet another by-product into new forms of value.[47]

Although cremation is becoming more efficient and clean burning, massive amounts of nonrenewable energy sources are used to maintain the furnace. The technology also generates carbon dioxide, noxious gases, and carcinogens. In response to these indications that cremation is wasteful and toxic, new flameless options neutralize harmful pathogens in organic material but remove the need for the corpse to undergo a polluting incinerator process. Resomation—also known as biocremation, water resolution, aquamation, bioliquefaction, and natural cremation—replaces the traditional use of fire with a water- and alkali-based method (alkaline hydrolysis).[48] Alkaline hydrolysis converts the tissue and cells of the human body into a watery solution of micromolecules, leaving a bone structure of mineral compounds, such as calcium and phosphates.[49] The corpse is placed into a pressurized steel vessel that heats it to approximately 350 degrees Fahrenheit under 150 pounds per square inch of pressure within a potassium hydroxide (lye) solution, breaking down flesh into nonhazardous salts, sugars, small peptides, and amino acids.[50] The effluent from the chemical process is sterile, contains no DNA, and can be discharged to the sewer system or a green space without further treatment. Metals present in the body prior to treatment can be recycled, while the skeletal remains are processed into white ash and returned to the deceased's family or guardians. The patented process normally takes two to three hours, similar to the average length of a flame-based cremation. Hailed by its purveyors as the responsible and ethical green choice, it allegedly produces one-third less greenhouse gas than incineration, consumes only 10 percent of the energy used during cremation, and allows for the safe separation of dental amalgam for disposal.[51] Even though recycling the liquid is not without significant controversy in the American context—particularly due to concerns about whether liquefaction violates respect for human remains and how to regulate the reincorporation of the solution into water treatment infrastructure—fourteen states have approved the use of the technology, with permits additionally implemented in California and pending approval in five more states.[52]

Just as the dead body is recycled for reuse—and the cremation process improved through more efficient and environmentally friendly technologies—the affirmation to green death, in all of these examples, reimagines the dead body within a feedback loop of economic and corporeal values—one in which the afterlife is not "the end" but a renewable material resource and bioremediation opportunity. Crematoria heat recycling in particular reveals this conceptual reinterpretation of the dead body from waste (for disposal) to reusable material and even "fuel" to warm the living (and maximize the life of living populations).[53] Extracting more from the dead body adds positive value under the sign of efficiency and exhibits a complex mix of ecological and commercial logics within the biopolitical governance of the dead.

Biopresence

At the intersection of environmental ethics and consumer rights, a sustainable death movement strives to mitigate the environmental impact and dispensation of human remains. Environmental concerns over the disposal of the dead challenge a number of death care practices and technologies, notably embalming and the toxicities generated by both conventional cremations and burials. Bioremediation can thus involve reimagining bodily decomposition as natural—"returning the dead body to nature"—and supporting land conservation through burial. We also observe new technologies and consumer products of commemoration that enable the expression of personal legacy in terms of environmental inheritance—in some cases, through converting the material remains of the dead into durable postmortem presence, from diamond rings to memorial trees or coral reefs. On the one hand, the sustainable death trend in biocultures of afterlife—exemplified by eco-friendly burials—rejects the commodification of death. On the other hand, we also see the proliferation of customized products and activities to enhance personal legacy. Greening death signals a shift in how we think about governing the dead body: this epistemological bioremediation advocates for the environmental benefits of the dead body and social responsibility of/for afterlife, yet also contradictorily may lead to intensified commercial and technical approaches to administering death.

For example, green burial options are making gains within American death care, honoring the dead through commemorating sustainability and redefining the corpse as a material input for land or nature. Rather than maintaining static biotic environments that emphasize containment and preservation, green burials or natural burials aim to "care for the dead with minimal ecological impact by eschewing embalming and non-biodegradable burial containers, vaults and liners."[54] They forward a radical "necro-ecological" agenda that revises assumptions about the nature of dead bodies and of the value of human decomposition to nature.[55] Contrary to popular repudiation of decay as a form of pollution, the human body—seen as a material, chemical, and biological component of the natural world—is integrated into an ecology of death. As a natural part of the ecosystem, corpses can generate biovalue through composting processes that benefit nature and living humans, in a kind of "cradle to grave" or "waste to food" intergenerational cycle.[56] The Urban Death Project, for example, proposes local corpse-reprocessing systems, wherein bodies are placed inside a three-story core and converted to compost with the help of aerobic decomposition and microbial activity.[57] According to the project website, it is "not simply a system for turning our bodies into soil-building material. It is also a space for contemplation of our place in the natural world, and a ritual to help us say goodbye to our loved ones by connecting us with the cycles of nature."[58] Moving from the architectural to the sartorial, the Infinity Burial Suit (called the Mushroom Death Suit in artist Jae Rhim Lee's original concept) is designed to be worn by the corpse for direct burial into the soil; the suit is embroidered with a special strain of fungi that, when buried, help to break down the body and remediate toxins that could contaminate the surrounding environment.[59] Lee also engineered an alternative embalming fluid—a liquid spore slurry—as well as Decompiculture Makeup, which, when applied, activates the mushrooms to develop and grow.

This interest in the ecology of death supports a land ethic—that the decomposition of the dead can contribute to conservation efforts—and new biopolitical and regulatory frameworks for American deathscapes that reward sustainable death best practices. The growing number of conservation burial grounds and cemetery nature preserves shows how human burial can dovetail with the need for land preservation and environmental stewardship. Traditional cemeteries increasingly allow for natural burial practices, and as of 2013, there were around thirty-seven certified green cemeteries in the United States; U.S. Funerals Online estimates the number of green burial cemeteries reached ninety-three in 2016.[60] The Green Burial Council—an independent nonprofit organization founded in 2005—established the nation's first certifiable standards for cemeteries, funeral providers, burial product manufacturers, and cremation facilities, positioning itself as arbiter of the green burial world (as both social movement and business opportunity).[61] Cemetery responses to these sustainability standards have ranged from hybrid burial grounds—conventional cemeteries that offer burial without a vault, container, or gravestone and that do not require embalming—to natural burial grounds that maintain energy-conserving and antitoxics protocols, integrated pest management, and natural landscaping compatible with regional ecosystems.[62]

With the median cost of a funeral in the United States reaching $7,181 in 2014, green burial can present significant economic savings, costing as little as $500.[63] Eco-friendly burial services might entail a home vigil and noninvasive techniques and materials to clean and preserve the dead body for a few days. Sustainability thus might refer to economic viability in addition to a land ethic or revaluation of human decay. A loosely knit do-it-yourself death movement is reclaiming various aspects of death, rejecting environmentally harmful measures to beautify the corpse, organizing "home death care" and personal funerals, and even arranging at-home backyard burial.[64] Ecological "death gear" options flourish alongside this trend of economically frugal disposal. A dynamic green burial market now supplies an outcropping of ecological coffins and shrouds that allow or even help the body to decay, ranging from a scaled-back traditional coffin with biodegradable glue, aqueous paint, and no metal to myriad artisanal caskets, cocoons, or eco-pods made of wicker, felt, cardboard, or paper mache. For example, California-based Eternity sells cardboard coffins for as little as $175, with wood-printed versions (cherry or pine) in soy ink for $320.[65] Among the Kinkaraco catalog of death shrouds, there are linen options for bodies as well as cremation remains, combined with biodegradable lowering devices, such as the TRU-GREEN BELIEVER in linen or the herbal-lined Botanika Deathspa.[66] Biodegradable urns have also emerged in the green death market, often mimicking natural forms and/or propagating plants, such as the ARKA acorn urn made from recycled paper and natural fibers and shaped like a large acorn; the sinkable biodegradable Shell Urn made from nontoxic food-grade recycled paper for burials on land or at sea; and the Bios Urn, which espouses the motto "There's life, after life" by integrating a pine seed inside of the vessel to support the growth of a tree following burial.[67]

The American demand for more customized and individually personalized forms of memorialization has spurred the transformation of material remains of the dead into new forms of postmortem "biopresence," from wearable "everlasting" art and commodities to environmental enhancements that redefine the relationship between human and nonhuman. Life-Gem offers "memorial diamonds" and commemorative wearables made from human ashes or a lock of human hair, not unlike Victorian-era death cult traditions of sculptures or jewelry made with human hair. The patented process extracts and purifies leftover carbon, and the resulting graphite is fashioned into a diamond, under intense heat and pressure.[68] Ashes can also be sterilized and mixed with tattoo ink for a uniquely subcutaneous commemoration of the deceased.[69] Other technologies create proprietary natures by integrating cremains or human DNA into other life-forms and postmortem cross-species interaction. While the use of human remains as a renewable building material is contentious, cremains are gaining ground as underwater infrastructure, namely, the interring or mixing of human ashes in "reef balls" for an aquatic-customized form of commemoration. For example, Eternal Reef is "a designed reef made of environmentally-safe cast concrete mixture that is used to create new marine habitats for fish and other forms of sea life."[70] The Eternal Reefs are then placed in a U.S.

Environmental Protection Agency–permitted ocean location, selected by the individual, friend, or family member to create public recreational reef structures. Small personal mementos can be included in the mix of the remains and concrete, along with ash from other family members or family pets. Reportedly, more than eighteen hundred Eternal Reefs are positioned off the coasts of Florida, South Carolina, North Carolina, Maryland, New Jersey, Texas, and Virginia.[71]

DNA memorial trees take this form of commemoration even further into the biosphere. An art venture formed by Shiho Fukuhara and Georg Tremmel, the project integrates human DNA into other life-forms. DNA "burials"—the transcoding of human DNA within the DNA of a tree or plant—have been hailed as the new space-saving transgenic tombstone in response to crowded cemeteries.[72] In collaboration with MIT Biology Lab affiliate/artist Joe Davies, the project—aptly named Biopresence—aims to produce a living memorial: "A tree that will look, grow, and behave like any other tree, but it would carry the biological information of a human."[73] Memorialization of the human takes on intensified bioengineered presence that challenges how humans relate to and bond with the dead and nature alike. At approximately $30,000, this extravagant *memento mori* fosters an unbounded posthuman "after life, but not as we know it," by treating personal legacy as literal environmental trace—a proprietary nature and right to the land as inheritance.[74]

Paradoxes of Greening Afterlives

U.S. biocultures of afterlife increasingly demonstrate the affirmation to green death and the dead body. As evidenced in the previous section, sustainability concerns and bioremediation are reinterpreting the material afterlife of the corpse. Such practices, however, do not take place outside of power relations: the administration of the dead intimately affirms life for some people or in some form while obscuring the deaths and deathly conditions of others. Foucault described biopolitical governance of the living as being "cut" by race—that racism is "a way of introducing a break into the domain of life that is under power's control: the break between what must live and what must die. . . . That is the first function of racism: to create caesuras within the biological continuum."[75] Various accounts of forms of death-in-life—abandonment or the slow violence of exposure— reveal that biopolitics is not merely about the managed optimization of life and livingness of human bodies but also about strategic allowances for death and qualifications of what or who counts as human, for the purposes of biosecurity, racial capitalism, colonial occupation, and, per Judith Butler's turn of phrase, what counts as a "grievable life."[76] The disposal and commemoration of human remains exemplify the materiality of power relations that operate in and through death. U.S. governance of the dead has entrenched racism in the landscape and inequitably treated the bodies of black people, American Indians, religious minorities, women, the poor, convicts, the homeless, and the mentally ill (to name a few). This reminds us, as we note in the chapter's second epigraph, "of the need constantly to situate reflections on our shared humanity in contexts of conquest and dispossession—as much of the corpse as of living subjects."[77] The governing of afterlife—particularly the material opportunities presented by the dead body—perpetuates inequalities and exclusions; life is affirmed as afterlife unevenly and contradictorily. If racism is about determining who is "let die" (i.e., caesuras in the population), then the material geographies of afterlife perpetuate and extend that cut: some people are made to live (more) even after death (through commemoration, through remaining present in some way), while others are denied bodily self-determination and/or social legacy. Thus we explore some of the potential hazards and costs of bioremediation and emerging sustainable death practices—of efforts to produce "no remains" and "biopresence" in the handling and disposal of the dead—and their effects on civil, consumer, and environmental rights. Examining some of the "death effects" of bioremediation—of efficient disposal or environmental legacy—galvanizes the basis for a material ethics of human remains.

First, the pursuit of "no remains," however laudable, risks further privatizing and obfuscating the labor of handling and disposing of the dead. Moreover, it may legitimate the status quo by making the dead body perform labor as infrastructure, gift, and so on—as the ultimate neoliberal renewable resource (i.e., even "dead" capital can be converted to biovalue). Intensified bioremediation of the dead body may paradoxically legitimate wasteful consumption and excess in American lifestyles by making disposal of the dead more efficient. This emphasis on efficiency not only promises profits or cost savings for involved companies (orthopedic implant recyclers, cremation providers, etc.) but also incurs desocializing effects, such as rapidly removing the dead body from everyday life, compressing grief and mourning into a shorter time span, and eliminating social gathering.[78] One of the contradictions of expanded technosocial relations with the material remains of the dead is that death potentially disappears from the social horizon as a collective activity: in other words, this could be the *social death of death*.[79] While there is increasingly a rich social networking of memorializing corpses in the digital realm as well as an expanding interest in home funerals and home-based death care, the social conditions of neoliberal self-care and austerity—set within a longer history of the secularization of death—also work to privatize the experience of death, reduce social responsibility for the administration of the dead, and potentially legitimate further cuts to governmental funding for death care and commemoration.[80]

Following earlier denunciations of the funeral trade for transforming the dead into highly profitable revenue streams via marketing techniques and synergies between the funeral firm and its products, restructuring of the "industry of death"—emphasizing sustainability, efficiency, and customization—may encourage religious and cultural diversification and meaningful experiences with dead bodies but also precipitate private stopgaps to the shrinkage of state support for death care and the eroded social safety net within the United States.[81] Sustainability in the context of death work may serve to greenwash austerity and further rationalize the corporatized infrastructure of the funeral industry itself. The commodification of the funeral process has advanced the growth of national funeral homes and the transnational corporatization of the funeral industry, resulting in death care industry monopolies that herald efficiencies as consumer gains.[82] Cheaper and faster handling of the dead body, however, may signal the extension of neoliberal self-care into death care—wherein the individual or family is privately expected to bear all responsibility for health in life *and* efficient disposal of the dead with minimal interruption to routine.

Second, there is an underbelly to governance of the dead/afterlife that emphasizes material reuse of the body and efficient disposal: the deeply historical and ongoing unequal burden of bioremediation of human remains. The continual expansion of the dead body as a tool in medicine and technology has had differential and often detrimental impacts on various minority groups in the United States and transnational geographies of clinical trial participants, who have borne medical abuse as living test subjects. Specific populations in the United States have been treated as exploitable resources and understood to be worth more as specimens. Indigenous human remains have been "preserved" by scientific institutions, universities, and museums, dispossessing American Indians of bodily sovereignty in death and property rights over the dead.[83] The bodies of African Americans have been imperiled repeatedly and inserted into medical experiments and treatments to support white life, including the grave robbing of black bodies to supply cadavers to medical schools, the appropriation of the Henrietta Lacks cell line, and biopiracy of body parts and genetic resources from enslaved bodies.[84]

These practices were not engaged in under the banner of "greening death" but as a means to extract resources and position some populations as expendable. While contemporary technologies that seek to extract more from the dead body and/or green death are said to add positive value under the sign of efficiency (i.e., recycling, waste reduction, charity, etc.), this historical context reveals that operations of repurposing at the level of the population can solidify inequalities. For example, efforts to donate organs and recycle body parts are shadowed by a global black market of organ trafficking as well as the influence of money in making claims on available organs.[85] The "efficient disposal" of whole populations—because they may be positioned as an economic drain—haunts organ donation and bioremediation more generally: there are clear tensions between their potential to affirm life positively but also to reproduce unequal relations of power. A crucial question, then, is *who benefits from bioremediation, and under what conditions?* The emphasis on reducing the wastefulness of disposal—and the imperative to be useful in death as in life—enriches the market and circuits of capital and civil infrastructure but also risks instrumentalizing the material afterlife of the body to secure and intensify neoliberal white nationalism (a point that we revisit later).

Third, choosing one's legacy is not an option for all. New forms of commemoration and sustainable burial may extend the reach of those people who are already privileged in relations of power: some people have a variety of choices that extend beyond life, while others face ongoing forms of exclusion in life and in death. The reduction of one's footprint in death through flameless cremation and new material expressions of legacy— whether memorial reefs or diamonds—are only accessible to those with financial standing and knowledge. The choice to leave no trace through natural burial also *risks dovetailing with and legitimating state violence orchestrated through austerity.* Many states in the United States have cut or eliminated funds that had assisted the poor in performing burial services, further reducing the social opportunity to determine the afterlife of the dead body. In response to escalating "funeral poverty"—the inability to pay for disposal of the dead—there are cases where the funeral home has offered to subsidize funeral services in exchange for accessing organs and facilitating donation.[86] Essentially, leaving no legacy is frequently the de facto reality for those who are subjected to state control and efficiencies in the disposal of the dead. In the United States, local or state governments typically bury the unclaimed bodies of the indigent, homeless people, undocumented immigrants, and "unknowns" in unmarked graves or potter's fields; increasingly, such bodies are cremated with no funeral.[87] An *environmental history of body disappearance* parallels that of biopresence and postmortem legacies, as starkly revealed by Puerto Rico's post–Hurricane Maria official death count of sixty-four, reportedly missing an excess of thousands of deaths. Following mass exposure of Puerto Ricans to the hurricane, the aftermath of incompetent, corrupt, and/or nonexistent aid extended by the U.S. government and its contractors has treated the island territory as a container of disposable citizens.[88] Discovery of a mass grave in southern Texas in 2014 uncovered the "expedient" disposal of bodies that perished in the border region: local policy allowed for contracted local funeral homes to dump hundreds of bodies of undocumented immigrants— who died while crossing the Texas–Mexico border—in trash bags, shopping bags, or no containers at all.[89] Such evidence of biopolitical expungement cannot be physically unearthed to remediate social consciousness in the case of countless fetal deaths, lowered fertility, and the imperiling of infant lives from lead poisoning in postindustrial Flint, Michigan. Quick-fix water provisions and the repeated cover-up made everyday municipal water infrastructure into the intergenerational "killing fields" of the majority– African American city.[90]

Fourth, the conversion of human remains into biopresence—whether as commercial commemorative objects or "donations to nature"—is a privileged act that obscures its contaminating effects. Efforts to return the corpse to nature endeavor to reverse the separation of death and the dead body from the environment.[91] Suzanne Kelly effectively summarizes the material–ecological impacts of this way of death: "over the past 150 years American death care has positioned human death outside of the cycles of nature, rendering a false story of death in which the dead body—as matter—is imagined as having no value to the more-than-human world."[92] Countering a long-standing prohibition against returning the dead body to the earth, sustainable death practices radically naturalize decay and decomposition of the body as necessary to life. However, such practices can involve a nostalgic recoding of the body as natural, when the living and dead body alike are sociotechnical in nature, with noncompostable and even hazardous body parts. Revaluing decomposition of the human corpse thus requires careful consideration of the relationship between nature and waste and the labor politics and material conditions of handling the dead. Corpses are part of the industrial landscape and generate hazards for those who live or work near places where dead bodies are processed, stored, and/ or converted into myriad new postmortal materials and commemorative objects.[93]

Finally, affirming the greenness of death—especially an environmental ethic that seeks to eradicate the human–nonhuman divide—fails to account for the ways bodily integrity remains, for many, compromised in life and in death and the ways such inequalities are historically sedimented in the landscape. American organization of deathscapes and burial practices historically have reflected and legitimated social status divisions and inequities that existed among the living. Cemetery landscapes expressed "the central paradox of equality and exclusivity": while advocating democracy and equality, many Americans went to great lengths to differentiate themselves in death, often organizing extravagant funeral processions and ostentatious monuments and accessories that contradicted the steady rationalization of the cemetery.[94] Furthermore, dead populations were arranged in ways that advocated existing discrimination and injustice: "what happened while you were alive applied to when you died."[95] African Americans and other racial and religious minority groups were frequently relegated to separate land areas or placed in the back or side of cemeteries, often left to disrepair, obscurity, and/or anonymity. Thus the governing of dead bodies—both at the biopolitical level and at the level of disciplining individual bodies—solidified social barriers *in*/*as* the inherited environment. While greening the disposal of one's body—to have a sustainable or green legacy—is viewed as a gift to nature, the aforementioned underside of this operation is further entrenchment of social position in life: only those privileged in life have control over their material traces after death. Moreover, naturalizing death may extend human domination by blurring the boundary between human and nature and further colonizing the natural world with human biopresence—a devastating intensification of white settler colonialism within the American landscape and its history of native genocide and Indian removal. Commemorative human DNA trees are potentially an extreme manifestation of this imperial impulse—an individualizing, narcissistic occupation of nature by those with privilege and means—and could signal a shift from social care for the dead to an individualistic "living on" in perpetuity, an amplified form of what Douglas James Davies has called "ecological immortality."[96]

Given the racialized environmental history of the United States and the violent legacy of human–nonhuman and person–thing social divisions in the landscape, contemporary efforts to make the disposal of the dead body more green and efficient may further rationalize "bad deaths" into obscurity—by rendering them invisible as "nature" or as the "natural corpse." Efforts to address injustices surrounding the end of life, such as material failures of the body that are the result of structural violence (e.g., racialized health risks and diseases), may be undercut by efficient "abandonment to nature." Greening the governance of death may further promulgate a race-neutral land ethic that blunts social responsibility for the dead by eclipsing important sociopolitical differences between a green cemetery and a forgotten mass grave. In other words, bioremediation—biopresence projects in particular—could further entrench American *necroecologies of whiteness.*[97]

State violence is sedimented in the landscape: where dead bodies are located and how human remains are treated are operations that secure the social–environmental and violent basis of white nationhood and nature in the United States. These necroecologies of whiteness include, for example, segregated cemeteries and the social abandonment of African American graves; the seizure and colonization of American Indian lands and burial grounds; the political violence of Jewish cemetery desecrations and those of other minorities; and the neglected, often unknown mass graves of those positioned as subordinate wards of the state or considered to be dangerous, in order to maintain the security of the (white) population.[98] Instrumentalizing nature as dumping ground works to absolve society of responsibility for the uneven care and opportunities experienced by different groups of people: such deaths look natural, as if no governance or power relations were involved. In such cases, nature does not preserve legacy but serves to depoliticize death, because human remains do not appear to signify or surface as the material ruins of injustice. In other words, green death risks further greenwashing an already stratified and racialized nature.

Death Justice: Material Ethics of Human Remains?

Affirming green death provides an opportunity to raise questions about the governance of dead bodies and deathscapes and to reimagine our ontologies and epistemologies of death—as a way to think anew about ethical relations, orientations, and actions toward life and death. This chapter has explored biocultures of afterlife—bioremediation efforts to create sustainability in the afterlife and the power relations of who or what materially remains after life; it has examined efforts to green death and their paradoxical consequences, contextualized with respect to overlapping environmental, consumer, and civil rights issues. The analysis was grounded in an understanding of the creation of value orchestrated by greening death: how the dead body is reconceived as a body able to be disciplined, to become a laboring and productive body even in death and a vehicle for value-generating environmental legacies. It also speculated on potentially deleterious effects and inequities related to forms of biopolitical administration of the dead, such as the intensification of anonymity and privatization of death under conditions of austerity; the uneven body politics and geographies of bioremediation—the underbelly of "mass disappearance" in relation to biopresence and memorialization; the ongoing imbrications of race and nature in the United States—"necroecologies of whiteness"—and violent extension of social death to the afterlife. Drawing on this critical–political ecology of death, we can ask how conduct for the dead and human remains might advance social justice.

As we have alluded to in the previous section, race- and class-based disparities in the control of human remains have led to cultural loss and community suffering as well as social protest and challenges to the death industry. Within the context of the United States' vast inequalities, death is also an opportunity to leave a material trace as a way to refuse anonymity. Whether one leaves a trace or not is a deeply political matter: it matters whether this is framed and experienced as a choice, and whether one has any control over the process and maintenance of the remains. Anonymous death might be desirable, but only as a choice. If one experienced limited freedom or agency in life, then the anonymity of death affirms that denial of subjectivity through expungement and abandonment of afterlife. Therefore, a material ethics of human remains that acknowledges that legacy—whether it be the conversion of the dead body to gift or energy, the anonymous decomposition of bodily remains as "food" to ecology, or the contestation over the dead as property—is always a material relation of

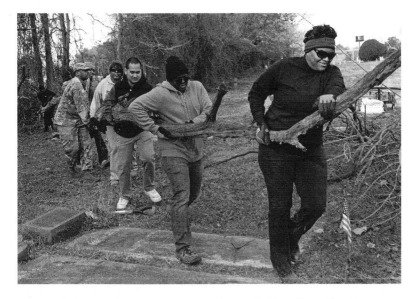

Figure 15. U.S. military and civilian community volunteers help restore the oldest and largest African American cemetery on the Virginia Peninsula, the Pleasant Shade Cemetery in Hampton, Virginia, 2017. U.S. Air Force photograph by Staff Sergeant Teresa J. Cleveland. The appearance of U.S. Department of Defense (DoD) visual information does not imply or constitute DoD endorsement.

power. Simultaneously, the idea of a remainder or residual trace animates the utopian possibility that those material relations of power are unfinished, indeterminate, and might be otherwise—and, at the very least, that social death-in-life may be countered with witnessing, nonanonymity, community reparations, reconciliation processes, or other forms of "living on" in death/afterlife.

By focusing on this material politics of human remains, we can explore ways to bridge environmental and social concerns through death care or, rather, *death justice*. Death justice efforts might inaugurate new geographies for our living together across the threshold that separates life and death. Traces of this exist, such as cemetery caretaking and maintenance programs that seek to reverse the neglect of African American burial grounds and, in doing so, cultivate reparative justice within U.S. environmental history.[99] Volunteer programs to bear witness to indigent burials advocate that everyone has the right to a social—not anonymous—death.[100] There are also examples of innovative cemeteries that open their gates to cross-programming, for example, to dog walkers who sign up to adopt a grave,

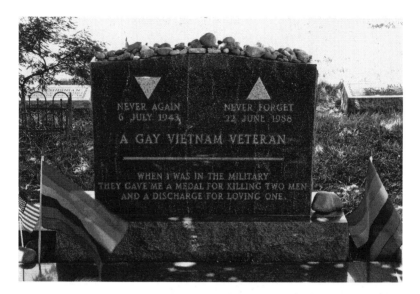

Figure 16. Vietnam War veteran Leonard P. Matlovich (1943–88) was the first gay service member to purposely out himself to the military to fight its ban on gays. His tombstone, intended as a memorial to all gay veterans, does not bear his name but reads "A Gay Vietnam Veteran" and "When I was in the military, they gave me a medal for killing two men and a discharge for loving one." The gravesite is located in Congressional Cemetery in Washington, D.C., and remains an icon. Photograph courtesy of F. Delventhal, reproduced under a Creative Commons Attribution 2.0 Generic (CC by 2.0) license, https://creativecommons.org/licenses/by/2.0/.

thereby integrating social responsibility for the remains of the dead with community stewardship and cross-species companionship.

Some cemeteries and columbaria support educational initiatives and lessons on activism within a national context of civil rights actions intimately connected to funeral gatherings.[101] People often leave wry commentary about social struggle in cemeteries that remain relevant today. In this sense, sustainability might refer to cultivating a heritage of intergenerational justice—as a charge to take up in the present—rather than efficiency, private eco-values, or technological mastery. The potential greening of the funeral industry may work to *un*-install embalming as a requirement of funeral director licensing and, in the process, advance economic justice by further diversifying a racially stratified profession—opening it up to communities and leaders of religious and cultural backgrounds that may prohibit embalming but seek to advocate their civil rights in or through death rites. Finally, efforts to recuperate and repatriate human and cultural remains build material support for legacies of self-determination, expand conviviality with the dead, and haunt the nation and institutions with evidence of their violent basis and reparation demands—from universities, archives, and museums to national parks.

These brief examples accept the living and the dead as cobelonging through different forms of recognition and care work with respect to human remains.[102] Death is an opportunity to address social failures and democratize the "good life" through enacting and sustaining more just relations with human remains. Advancing the social recognition of death and stewardship of material remains challenges us to imagine how to act on behalf of a "good death"—as something more than the negation of life or failure to live—as an incitement to overhaul death's governance and, in so doing, deathly social conditions in life. For if we do not treat the dead well, what hope is there for the living?[103]

Coda

Endure

Admittedly, "death informing life" will seem counter-intuitive or even insane to us because, as Foucault has claimed, in the last two centuries we no longer properly speak *of death. Discourses on death are as forgotten and disavowed as the nameless and innumerable deaths themselves. In the last two centuries, Foucault argues, political and sovereign discourses have focused instead on life. Life has eclipsed death.*

—Stuart Murray, "Thanatopolitics"

A politics of care engages much more than a moral stance; it involves affective, ethical, and hands-on agencies of practical and material consequence.

—María Puig de la Bellacasa, *Matters of Care*

Life-making remains the dominant political paradigm in contemporary U.S. biocultures today, even as it is increasingly inflected and conditioned by neoliberal rationalities. Life is maximized, optimized, and prolonged via a range of strategies and technologies that *affirm life*. Within this paradigm, life is framed as that which must be constantly tended and relentlessly avowed: death must be disavowed. Such harnessing of life is promoted as a universal good, a "virtual cosmology for us, its subjects."[1]

Our central claim throughout this analysis, however, has been that life-making in U.S. biocultures operates as a regulatory politics of affirmation that intimately governs the daily existence and possible futures of individuals and communities. More than this, life-making can be—and is often—deadly. The underside of the "make live" imperative of biopolitics—where subjects must be *made to live*—entails contemporaneous operations of abandonment, negligence, and oversight: this is the "let die" function of biopolitics. We see this operating even with the affirmation to green, where life is affirmed as afterlife, at the same time as the lives/deaths of many are disclaimed, renounced, and made invisible. Death, then, does not disappear in this politics focused on life. Rather, it loses the spectacular ritual character (of "make die") that it had under sovereign premodern power and is instead hidden away—often in plain sight, *everywhere*. Structural and ideological workings of race, class, gender, sexuality, and other geopolitical specificities condition the operations of biopolitics. As Didier Fassin has noted, then, "biopolitics has consequences in terms of inequalities [and] governmentality conveys the disparities in the quantity and quality of life."[2] Not all lives and forms of life are fostered equally, and death's disavowal clearly does not extend to all. Some deaths don't even register *as* deaths. As we have explored, the very operations of "making live" can obscure ongoing deaths, can create deadly conditions, and can produce death and/or death effects. This is deadly life-making.

If death is folded into life-making, it seems essential that we cultivate a politics that is attentive to death—that can speak in the name of death and the innumerable lives imperiled or lost in biopolitical (and then often disciplinary) life-making operations. Such a politics would insist that death and forms of death-in-life are recognized as products of life-making practices and rhetoric. It would also act as a possible platform from which to affirm a different ethics or way of living (and dying). Throughout the preceding chapters, we have explored a range of strategies, tactics, techniques, and practices that enact such a politics. Collectively, they highlight that another kind of life is possible: "life is not only a question of politics from the outside in but should also be [and *is*] seized from the inside, in the flesh of the everyday experiences of social agents."[3]

In one incantation, this seizing of politics from the inside—in the flesh—can be viewed as endurance, understood as the capacity of something to last or to withstand wear and tear: it is the fact of enduring a difficult process without giving away. To endure is to remain in existence and, in the context of our analysis here, to find ways to *live on* despite the ongoing imperiling of life's continuance.[4] In another incantation, we might understand such a politics as being predicated on the notion of survival. Following the framing offered by Jacques Derrida, survival (which he also referred to as "living on," in a 1981 essay of the same name) is that which disrupts the distinction between biological life and life as an existential phenomenon: "survival is a complication of the opposition death-life."[5] In Derrida's formulation, survival complicates this dualism because it is at once the "unconditional affirmation" of life (continuing to live—understood here quite differently from triumphant biopolitical affirmation) and the "hope of 'surviving' through the traces left for the living."[6] Stemming from this line of thought, we could conceive the political enactments addressed in preceding chapters as tactics that simultaneously *affirm other ways to live now*—in ways that counteract dominant affirmations of life and their deadly effects—and insist on leaving enduring traces of their efforts that would alter the future social terrain. Through such tactics, people and collectives "transform their physical life into a political instrument or a moral resource or an affective expression" that demands change in relation to our biofutures.[7]

To expand, such demands for change might be seen to rest on three interrelated factors, which we have examined throughout *Deadly Biocultures* and that point out potential ways forward. First, it seems necessary *not* to turn away from death but, rather, to sit with sorrow and mourn the forestalling of life that occurs all around us. "It is, perhaps, a time to mourn together, to keep a vigil, and to invent new symbols that will come to occupy the spaces of indescribable loss, the spaces of everyday life, to make this loss and this life somehow livable."[8] Mourning, here, is a way to refuse death's disavowal and instead insist on the recognition of death's presence in life. Such mourning must not be viewed as simply passive. Instead, it can engender an elegiac politics—which enables representation for what are often lives lived *in* elegy. As S. Lochlain Jain has noted, "elegiac politics yearns to account for loss, grief, betrayal, and the connections between economic profits, disease, and death in a culture that is affronted by mortality."[9]

Second, this mourning must be matched with insistent critique. Speaking specifically in relation to racial inequities (though we can extend this idea to the various forms of death and deathly effects we have analyzed here), Katherine McKittrick has noted that critique requires that we "dwell on the particularities of injustice anew" to "attend to violence and sadness and the struggle for life."[10] She warns, however, that the very process of naming "let die" operations in academic criticism risks routinizing and re-producing practices that continue to mark the same people for death. Instead, we require examinations of and support for practices that actively contest the status quo and reinvent creative strategies of "living on"—those in existence already as well as more speculative projects.[11] Another way to think of critique is to adopt Foucault's understanding, where critique operates as "an instrument for those who fight, those who resist and refuse what is. . . . It is a challenge directed to what is."[12] For Foucault, a general characterization of critique is "the art of not being governed quite so much."[13] To critique the deadly operations of dominant affirmations of life in relation to biomedicine—and the extension of biomedical logics into everyday life—entails contesting pervasive regimes of health; questioning forms of governance that delimit how health, well-being, life, and death can be understood; and creating openings for alternative biofutures. We have analyzed the normativizing conventions and intimate governing functions of affirmations to hope, target, thrive, secure, and green—and those critical practices that wage against such affirmations. What other kinds of insurgent critique might be—or are—staged in these and other biocultural arenas?

Finally, alongside refusing death's disavowal through mourning and staging insurgent critique, it seems imperative that we attend to ourselves and one another through new and expansive forms of care. In the preceding chapters, we have explored a range of creative practices of care that push against biopolitical logics at work within particular biocultural spheres in late liberalism. Indeed, the necessary political rejoinder to deadly life-making appears as an ontology of care—where *care denotes the ethical practice and enactment of critique* (that we outline above) and efforts to repair our social sphere so that we can live and die as well as possible.[14] An ontology of care "expose[s] how neoliberal biopolitics makes live and lets die—how it kills in the name of life, and relies on the differential production of corporeal vulnerability and death as our *modus vivendi*."[15] Care acknowledges and responds to the biopolitical (and disciplinary) production of death, through recognition, refusal, and tending to life otherwise. Through care we might enable new socialities, where life is cultivated and affirmed in different ways: as a communal rather than individual pursuit; as that which enables co-belonging across thresholds (that separate within life and between life and death) and that bridge autonomy and relationality; and where dependency, interdependency, and shared vulnerability are foregrounded rather than denigrated.[16] This ontology of care is—and will continue to be—a difficult path, particularly when divisiveness and vulnerability are produced, maintained, mobilized, and exploited as core governing tactics of neoliberal biopolitics. To labor against deadly life-making, then, will ultimately require vigilance in relentlessly centering death in counterpolitics and practices. It will require that death and the deadly effects of governing logics and strategies inform how we will endure and *live on*.

Notes

Introduction

1. Nikolas Rose describes "late liberalism" as a shift in state responsibility from a role that grants and guarantees rights to one that ensures that the market operates through law and order. Describing this shift, he states, "The relation of the state and the people was to take a different form: the former would maintain the infrastructure of law and order; the latter would promote individual and national well-being by their responsibility and enterprise." See Nikolas Rose, *Powers of Freedom: Reframing Political Thought* (Cambridge: Cambridge University Press, 1999), 139. This era entails the shrinkage of the government's social functions under the auspices of "freeing" the economy and a new set of government rationalities and practices—commonly referred to as "neoliberal"—that aim to produce subjects that are self-enterprising, productive, autonomous individuals. These neoliberal rationalities do not so much roll back the state as they create widespread institutional/policy, cultural, and legal conditions that optimize the economy through the entrepreneurship of individuals, families, firms, and so on. According to Wendy Brown, neoliberalism is "a governing rationality through which everything is 'economized' and in a very specific way: human beings become market actors and nothing but, every field of activity is seen as a market, and every entity (whether public or private, whether person, business, or state) is governed as a firm.... Neoliberalism construes even non–wealth generating spheres—such as learning, dating, or exercising—in market terms, submits them to market metrics, and governs them with market techniques and practices. Above all, it casts people as human capital who must constantly tend to their own present and future value." Refer to Wendy Brown, interviewed by Timothy Shenk, "Booked #3: What Exactly Is Neoliberalism?," April 2, 2015, https://www.dis sentmagazine.org/blog/booked-3-what-exactly-is-neoliberalism-wendy-brown -undoing-the-demos (accessed March 26, 2018).

2. Nikolas Rose, *The Politics of Life Itself: Biomedicine, Power, and Subjectivity in the Twenty-First Century* (Princeton, N.J.: Princeton University Press, 2007), 25. Rose continues, "From official discourses of health promotion through narratives of the experience of disease and suffering in the mass media, to popular discourses on dieting and exercise, we see an increasing stress on personal

reconstruction through acting on the body in the name of a fitness that is simultaneously corporeal and psychological" (26).

3. Biomedicialization temporally follows an earlier period of medicalization—which marks social transformation of the last half of the twentieth century wherein aspects of life (previously considered outside the domain of medicine) became folded into an expanding arena of medicine and construed as "medical problems." Refer to Adele E. Clarke, Laura Mamo, Jennifer R. Fishman, Janet K. Shim, and Jennifer Ruth Fosket, "Biomedicalization: Technoscientific Transformations of Health, Illness, and U.S. Biomedicine," *American Sociological Review* 68 (2003): 161.

4. Clarke et al., 162. Also see Adele E. Clarke, Laura Mamo, Jennifer Ruth Fosket, Jennifer R. Fishman, and Janet K. Shim, eds., *Biomedicalization: Technoscience, Health, and Illness in the U.S.* (Durham, N.C.: Duke University Press, 2010).

5. We argue that affirmation is central to biopolitics and is regulatory and normative. As we explain later in this introduction, this approach is different than that of "affirmative biopolitics," which positions itself as a critique of the "negative" side of biopolitics; affirmation by this account refers to the reclaiming of life from governmental apparatuses. See, for example, Roberto Esposito's trilogy *Bios: Biopolitics and Philosophy* (Minneapolis: University of Minnesota Press, 2008), *Communitas: The Origin and Destiny of Community* (Stanford, Calif.: Stanford University Press, 2009), and *Immunitas: The Protection and Negation of Life* (Cambridge, Mass.: Polity, 2011).

6. Thomas Lemke, *Foucault, Governmentality, and Critique* (New York: Routledge, 2016), 13.

7. Michel Foucault, *The History of Sexuality: Vol. 1. An Introduction,* trans. Robert Hurley (New York: Vintage Books, 1990), 136. Biopower is distinct from an earlier form of power that Foucault calls *sovereign power.* "Sovereignty took life and let live." It was a form of power that was negating, legislative, prohibitive, censoring, and homogenous. See Michel Foucault, *Society Must Be Defended: Lectures at the Collège de France 1975–1976,* trans. David Macey (New York: Picador, 2003), 247. Thus, where sovereign power operated in a repressive sense, modern biopower is normalizing and productive. This is not to say that forms of sovereign power are not still exercised. It recedes, however, because "life more than law became the issue of political struggles." Foucault, *History of Sexuality,* 144.

8. Éric Darier, "Foucault and the Environment: An Introduction," in *Discourses of the Environment,* ed. Eric Darier (Oxford: Blackwell, 1999), 22.

9. Thomas Lemke, *Biopolitics: An Advanced Introduction* (New York: New York University Press, 2011), 37.

10. Foucault, *Society Must Be Defended,* 241.

11. Foucault, 254.

12. Note that, according to Foucault, discipline emerged prior to biopolitics. Disciplinary power, as Foucault tells us, began to take hold in the late seventeenth and early eighteenth centuries (whereas bioplitics emerged in the second half of the eighteenth century): he links discipline to the rise of industrialization and capitalism. Per Deborah Cook, "Foucault describes the relation between power—the disciplinary colonization of the body—and the economy as both reciprocal and complex." See Cook, "'Is Power Always Secondary to the Economy?' Foucault and Adorno on Power and Exchange," *Foucault Studies,* no. 20 (2015): 186.

13. Michel Foucault, *Discipline and Punish: The Birth of the Prison,* trans. Alan Sheridan (New York: Vintage Books, 1995), 170.

14. In contradistinction to the sovereign and juridical model of power as repressive (i.e., taking life) and an "oppressive" understanding of subjection—such as seizure or punishment—this model of power targets the body to produce certain kinds of subjectivity that are obedient to normalizing technologies. These normalizing technologies enlist norms that are gendered, racialized, corporealized, medicalized, militarized, and so forth—that call forth/interpellate subjects as such. Note that discipline does not equate to "passivity" but, rather, the process of subjection that involves, in Judith Butler's words, "the principle of regulation according to which a subject is formulated or produced." Refer to Foucault, *Discipline and Punish,* 29; Judith Butler, *The Psychic Life of Power: Theories in Subjection* (Stanford, Calif.: Stanford University Press, 1997), 84.

15. Foucault, *Society Must Be Defended,* 242.

16. Foucault, 242–43. Also see Cook, "Is Power Always Secondary to the Economy?," 187. As Thomas Lemke has noted, "They [discipline and biopolitics] are not independent entities but define each other. Accordingly, discipline is not a form of individualization that is applied to already existing individuals, but rather it presupposes a multiplicity. Similarly, population constitutes the combination and aggregation of individualized patterns of existence *to a new political form.* It follows that 'individual' and 'mass' are not extremes but rather . . . simultaneously aims at the control of the human as individual body and at the human as species." Lemke, *Biopolitics,* 37–38, emphasis added.

17. In our reading of Foucault, it is biopolitical power that is more thoroughly focused on "life"—and that marks "power's hold over life." Foucault, *Society Must Be Defended,* 239. Indeed, Foucault distinguishes between "the regulatory technology of life [biopolitics] and the disciplinary technology of the body" (249). Biopolitics, he tells us, "is centered not upon the body but upon life" (249). This is not to say that disciplinary power does not come to concern itself with life-making: as we note, precisely because biopolitics embeds itself within discipline, disciplinary operations often work in line with biopolitical operations to "make live." Both discipline and biopolitics, however, ultimately compose the power over life that Foucault names biopower. See Lemke, *Biopolitics,* 36.

18. Foucault explains how the population becomes the subject and object of power focused on "improving life." Processes of "regularization" work to foster certain kinds of life, regularize those lives, and massify individual bodies and selves for governing in order to then foster and extract the capacities of that collective "life" or body of the population. Refer to Foucault, *Society Must Be Defended*, 248.

19. Pasquale Pasquino, "Theatrum Politicum: The Genealogy of Capital—Police and the State of Prosperity," in *The Foucault Effect: Studies in Governmentality*, ed. Graham Burchell, Colin Gordon, and Peter Miller (Chicago: University of Chicago Press, 1991), 113.

20. Foucault, *Society Must Be Defended*, 241.

21. Stuart J. Murray, "Thanatopolitics: On the Use of Death for Mobilizing Political Life," *Polygraph: An International Journal of Politics and Culture* 18 (2006): 197.

22. Stuart J. Murray, "Care of the Self: Biotechnology, Reproduction, and the Good Life," *Philosophy, Ethics, and Humanities in Medicine* 2, no. 6 (2007), http://www.peh-med.com/content/2/1/6 (accessed November 28, 2014).

23. For more on "social death," see Orlando Patterson, *Slavery and Social Death: A Comparative Study* (Cambridge, Mass.: Harvard University Press, 1982); for a discussion of "premature death," see Ruth Wilson Gilmore, *Golden Gulag: Prisons, Surplus, Crisis, and Opposition in Globalizing California* (Berkeley: University of California Press, 2007); and for more on "slow death," see Lauren Berlant, "Slow Death (Sovereignty, Obesity, Lateral Agency)," *Critical Inquiry* 33, no. 4 (2007): 754–80.

24. Also see below, where we further refine how we address death within a life-making power—delineating our approach from other accounts of operations of death in the politics of life.

25. Foucault, *Society Must Be Defended*, 256.

26. Melinda Cooper, *Life as Surplus: Biotechnology and Capitalism in the Neoliberal Era* (Seattle: University of Washington Press, 2008), 8–11.

27. While our analysis remains primarily tethered to the national scale, U.S. biocultures are transnational and necessitate further examination from postcolonial perspectives and geographies. This ranges from the outsourcing of clinical trials to the Global South, where bodies bear collateral damage in support of U.S. life-making efforts, to the U.S. reliance on immigrant labor to maintain key areas of the national health care system and various health industries and infrastructure, such as care for the elderly. For examples of scholarship on the former, see Adriana Petryna, *When Experiments Travel: Clinical Trials and the Global Search for Human Subjects* (Princeton, N.J.: Princeton University Press, 2009); Susan Craddock, "Drug Partnerships and Global Practices," *Journal of Health and Place* 18, no. 3 (2012): 481–89; and Kaushik Sunder Rajan, ed., *Lively Capital:*

Biotechnologies, Ethics, and Governance in Global Markets (Durham, N.C.: Duke University Press, 2012).

28. Note that our methodology predominantly relies on discursive analysis, including that of practices; the book is not an ethnographic account of practitioners.

29. Throughout this book, we use the terms *white* and *black* to denote broad racial oppositions constructed in Western (post)-Enlightenment logic systems rather than distinct categories. Where we do capitalize certain racial or ethnic categories, it is to mark those groups that are differentiated through biomedical and state-based practices (such as the census). And while such categories remain important—in order for groups to make demands on the state/social sphere— they obfuscate the diversity within groups and are also necessarily constructed in historically and geographically specific ways.

30. Nikolas Rose and Carlos Novas, "Biological Citizenship," in *Global Assemblages: Technology, Politics, and Ethics as Anthropological Problems,* ed. Aihwa Ong and Stephen J. Collier (Malden, Mass.: Blackwell, 2005), 439–63. Adriana Petryna first used this term in *Life Exposed: Biological Citizens after Chernobyl* (Princeton, N.J.: Princeton University Press, 2002).

31. Paul Rabinow, "Artificiality and Enlightenment: From Sociobiology to Biosociality," in *Essays on the Anthropology of Reason,* 91–111 (Princeton, N.J.: Princeton University Press, 1996).

32. Catherine Waldby, "Stem Cells, Tissue Cultures, and the Production of Biovalue," *Health* 6, no. 3 (2002): 310.

33. Waldby, 310.

34. Rose, *Politics of Life Itself,* 32. Also see Carlos Novas and Nikolas Rose, "Genetic Risk and the Birth of the Somatic Individual," *Economy and Society* 29, no. 4 (2000): 485–513.

35. Kaushik Sunder Rajan, *Biocapital: The Constitution of Postgenomic Life* (Durham, N.C.: Duke University Press, 2006); Melinda Cooper, *Life as Surplus.* Also see Catherine Waldby and Robert Mitchell, *Tissue Economies: Blood, Organs, and Cell Lines in Late Capitalism* (Durham, N.C.: Duke University Press, 2006), and Clarke et al., *Biomedicalization.*

36. Our biocultural approach draws on the insights and earlier institutional efforts of Lennard J. Davis, who advocated for biocultural literacy across publics to address complex questions of life and death. Bringing together the disciplines of science, technology, medicine, and the humanities, Davis and Project Biocultures at the University of Illinois–Chicago innovatively created a "biocultural studies" platform for issues concerning the body, identity, bio/technology, history, and culture. See Davis, "Life, Death, and Biocultural Literacy," *The Chronicle Review* 52, no. 18 (2006), http://www.lennarddavis.com/downloads/lifedeathand bioculture.pdf (accessed May 23, 2019). Notably, Rajshree Chandra also uses the

term *biocultures* in her work on the politics of genetic resources and new biotic properties and rights, *The Cunning of Rights: Law, Life, Biocultures* (New Delhi: Oxford University Press, 2016). Samantha Frost deploys the term to denote how humans become cultured within the particularities of their material, social, and symbolic worlds in *Biocultural Creatures: Toward a New Theory of the Human* (Durham, N.C.: Duke University Press, 2016). As noted earlier in this introduction, we use the term to describe the various ways biomedical logics and rationalities extend into broader society (escape biomedical confines) and become incorporated into social practices and individual self-formation and governance. We also utilize biocultures as a methodology.

37. See, e.g., Esposito, *Bios: Biopolitics and Philosophy.*

38. Refer to Giorgio Agamben, *Homo Sacer: Sovereign Power and Bare Life* (Stanford, Calif.: Stanford University Press, 1998). On death and biopolitics in "societies of control," see Michael Hardt and Antonio Negri, *Empire* (Cambridge, Mass.: Harvard University Press, 2000), and Michael Hardt and Antonio Negri, *Commonwealth* (Cambridge, Mass.: Harvard University Press, 2009).

39. Achille Mbembe, "Necropolitics," *Public Culture* 15, no. 1 (2003): 14. For a wide-ranging investigation of "queer necropolitics" in "everyday death worlds"— an approach that overlaps with that of this volume—refer to the anthology by Jin Haritaworn, Adi Kuntsman, and Silvia Posocco, eds., *Queer Necropolitics* (New York: Routledge, 2014).

40. Foucault, *History of Sexuality,* 136. Stuart Murray has argued that within this form of power, "life must be avowed; death disavowed. Life must be made; death is neither made nor unmade." Murray, "Thanatopolitics," 197. This is a relative passivity then. As Berlant has noted, Foucault shifts from a focus on "scenes of *control* over individual life and death under sovereign regimes and refocuses on the dispersed *management* of the biological threat posed by certain populations to the reproduction of the normatively framed general good life of a society." Berlant, "Slow Death," 756.

41. Anne Pollock, *Medicating Race: Heart Disease and Durable Preoccupations with Difference* (Durham, N.C.: Duke University Press, 2012).

42. Grace Kyungwon Hong, *Death Beyond Disavowal: The Impossible Politics of Difference* (Minneapolis: University of Minnesota Press, 2015).

43. Patterson, *Slavery and Social Death.*

44. Lisa Marie Cacho, *Social Death: Racialized Rightlessness and the Criminalization of the Unprotected* (New York: New York University Press, 2012), quote in book summary blurb.

45. Berlant, "Slow Death," 764.

46. Henry A. Giroux, "Reading Hurricane Katrina: Race, Class, and the Biopolitics of Disposability," *College Literature* 33, no. 3 (2006): 171–96; Matthew Sparke, "Austerity and the Embodiment of Neoliberalism as Ill-Health: Towards

a Theory of Biological Sub-citizenship," *Social Science and Medicine* 187 (2017): 287–95; Gilmore, *Golden Gulag,* 28.

47. As Chih-Chen Trista Lin, Claudio Minca, and Meghann Ormond have argued, "affirmative biopolitics is broadly understood . . . as a way to theorize how new/different ways of living and forms of life have the potential to transform or resist modes of dominance over, or negation of, life. Thinking in terms of affirmative biopolitics means considering the generative 'force' in the so-called 'politics of life,' whereby the power of life may be reclaimed from governmental apparatuses." See Lin et al., "Affirmative Biopolitics: Social and Vocational Education for Quechua Girls in the Postcolonial 'Affectsphere' of Cusco, Peru," *Environment and Planning D: Society and Space* 36, no. 5 (2018), https://doi.org/10.1177/0263775817753843 (accessed March 26, 2018). For variations on affirmative biopolitics, see Esposito's work, whose main point of reference for an affirmative biopolitics is bodies that oppose the external domination of life processes, and Rosi Braidotti, *The Posthuman* (Cambridge: Polity Press, 2013).

48. For an overview of new materialisms, refer to Diana Coole and Samantha Frost, "Introducing the New Materialisms," in *New Materialisms: Ontology, Agency, and Politics,* ed. Diana Coole and Samantha Frost, 1–43 (Durham, N.C.: Duke University Press, 2010). Also refer to Stacy Alaimo's reflexive contributions to new materialist scholarship, such as her article "Sustainable This, Sustainable That: New Materialisms, Posthumanism, and Unknown Futures," *PMLA* 127, no. 3 (2012): 558–64. Also see Eugene Thacker, *After Life* (Chicago: University of Chicago Press, 2010).

49. Lee Edelman, *No Future: Queer Theory and the Death Drive* (Durham, N.C.: Duke University Press, 2004).

50. Alastair Hunt and Stephanie Youngblood, eds., *Against Life* (Evanston, Ill.: Northwestern University Press, 2016).

1. Hope

1. See, e.g., Mary Zournazi, *Hope: New Philosophies for Change* (Annandale, Australia: Pluto Press, 2002).

2. See the Convoy of Hope website at http://www.convoyofhope.org/ (accessed November 28, 2014).

3. Thus we focus here on the governing logics of hope rather than on forms of resistance to such governing. Our interest is to explore how hope is deployed to invite individuals to think about themselves in particular ways and respond to biomedical facts and treatments according to dominant biomedical discourses. This is not to say that there are not myriad ways in which individuals and collectives challenge or reject such forms of governing.

4. Our use of the term *militarized* refers to the general process by which hope has been imbued with martial qualities and practiced across a range of scales for the purposes of security, namely, the organization of life—of institutions, knowledge, and social relations—according to the imperatives of national defense or individual survival, including everyday, banal neoliberal processes that naturalize social inequities and seek to contain social conflict by bounding spaces and bodies.

5. For an instructive overview of the affective turn, refer to Ruth Leys, "The Turn to Affect: A Critique," *Critical Inquiry* 37, no. 3 (2011): 434–72. Within contemporary theory, affect is understood in a range of ways: as immanent to the subject, the prediscursive or biologized substrate; as that which escapes reason, rationality, and intention; as nonsignifying, formless intensity or vital energy in excess of the human and the social. For example, Eric Shouse, referring to Brian Massumi's theory of affect, states that "an affect is a nonconscious experience of intensity; it is a moment of unformed and unstructured potential." Shouse, "Feeling, Emotion, Affect," *M/C Journal: A Journal of Media and Culture* 8, no. 6 (2005), http://journal.media-culture.org.au/0512/03-shouse.php (accessed November 28, 2014). Affect is understood to occur below the threshold of consciousness and cognition, independent of signification and meaning. It is also seen as "proceeding *directly* from the body—and indeed *between bodies*—without the interference or limitations of consciousness, or representation: For this reason, its force is, strictly speaking, pre-personal." Constantina Papoulias and Felicity Callard, "Biology's Gift: Interrogating the Turn to Affect," *Body and Society* 16, no. 1 (2010): 35. Such a prepersonal possibility between bodies (or material intensities) is considered to be the space from which a dynamic politics can emerge: "an essentially dynamic, self-organizing biology/nature is presented as the guarantor for an emancipatory and creative politics" (Papoulias and Callard, 49). In contradistinction to the emphasis on affect's immanence in much contemporary scholarship, our approach emphasizes the nonimmanent dynamics of affect—its social–relational–material functions.

6. Clare Hemmings, "Invoking Affect," *Cultural Studies* 19, no. 5 (2005): 565, emphasis added.

7. Mary J. Del Vecchio Good, B. J. Good, C. Schaffer, and S. E. Lind, "American Oncology and the Discourse of Hope," *Culture, Medicine, and Psychiatry* 14, no. 1 (1990): 59–79; Sarah Franklin, *Embodied Progress: A Cultural Account of Assisted Conception* (Abingdon, U.K.: Routledge, 1997); Tiago Moreira and Paolo Palladino, "Between Truth and Hope: On Parkinson's Disease, Neurotransplantation and the Production of the 'Self,'" *History of the Human Sciences* 18, no. 3 (2005): 55–82; Carlos Novas, "The Political Economy of Hope: Patients' Organizations, Science and Biovalue," *BioSocieties* 1, no. 3 (2006): 289–305. On Nik Brown's work, see "Ordering Hope: Representations of Xenotransplantation—An

Actant/Actor Network Theory Account" (PhD diss., Lancaster University, 1998); "Hope against Hype: Accountability in Biopasts, Presents and Futures," *Science Studies* 16, no. 2 (2003): 3–21; "Shifting Tenses: Reconnecting Regimes of Truth and Hope," *Configurations* 13, no. 3 (2005): 331–55; and "Shifting Tenses—From 'Regimes of Truth' to 'Regimes of Hope,'" SATSU Working Paper 30 (2006), http://www.york.ac.uk/media/satsu/documents-papers/Brown-2006-shifting.pdf. See also Cheryl Mattingly's work on hope as a narrative phenomenology of practice for families with critically ill children in *The Paradox of Hope: Journeys through a Clinical Borderland* (Berkeley: University of California Press, 2010).

8. We use the term *truth* here in the Foucauldian sense, to refer to a regime comprising types of discourse that an individual society "accepts and makes function as true." See Michel Foucault, "Truth and Power," in *Power/Knowledge: Selected Interviews and Other Writings, 1972–1977,* ed. Colin Gordon, trans. Colin Gordon, Leo Marshall, John Mepham, and Kate Soper, 109–33 (New York: Pantheon Books, 1980), esp. 131.

9. Nikolas Rose, *The Politics of Life Itself: Biomedicine, Power, and Subjectivity in the Twenty-First Century* (Princeton, N.J.: Princeton University Press, 2007); Adele E. Clarke, Laura Mamo, Jennifer Ruth Fosket, Jennifer R. Fishman, and Janet K. Shim, eds., *Biomedicalization: Technoscience, Health, and Illness in the U.S.* (Durham, N.C.: Duke University Press, 2010).

10. Susan Sontag, *Illness as Metaphor and AIDS and Its Metaphors* (New York: Picador, 1989).

11. Sontag, 17.

12. Robert N. Proctor, *Cancer Wars: How Politics Shapes What We Know and Don't Know about Cancer* (New York: Basic Books, 1996).

13. The beginnings of the modern era of cancer chemotherapy can be directly traced to the development and application of chemical warfare during World War I. For more on the linkages between the military–industrial complex and cancer control and treatment, refer to Bruce A. Chabner and Thomas G. Roberts, "Chemotherapy and the War on Cancer," *Nature Reviews Cancer* 5 (January 2005): 65–72; Sarah Hazell, "Mustard Gas—From the Great War to Frontline Chemotherapy," *Cancer Research UK "Science"* (blog), August 27, 2014, http://scienceblog.cancerresearchuk.org/2014/08/27/mustard-gas-from-the-great-war-to-frontline-chemotherapy/ (accessed July 21, 2016); John E. Fenn and Robert Udelsman, "First Use of Intravenous Chemotherapy Cancer Treatment: Rectifying the Record," *Journal of the American College of Surgeons* 212, no. 3 (2011): 413–17, http://www.journalacs.org/article/S1072-7515(10)01211-1/ (accessed July 21, 2016); "War Gases Tried in Cancer Therapy: Army Branch Joins Research Groups in Study of Using Nitrogen Blister Chemicals," *New York Times,* October 6, 1946, https://www.nytimes.com/1946/10/06/archives/war-gases-tried-in-cancer-therapy-army-branch-joins-research-groups.html (accessed July 21, 2016);

Novogen, "The Future of Cancer Therapy," January 2015, http://www.novogen
.com/pdf/cytotoxiChemotherapy.pdf (accessed July 21, 2016).

14. For Nikolas Rose, biocitizenship marks "all those citizenship projects that
have linked their conceptions of citizens to beliefs about the biological existence
of human beings, as individuals, as men and women, as families and lineages, as
communities, as populations and race, and as species." Rose, *Politics of Life Itself*,
132. What we go on to show, however, is that biocitizenship does not always
take nationalized form. Indeed, as Rose has argued, in the contemporary era,
it involves medical knowledge of one's "condition," a sense of belonging with
others who share that condition, and a heightened sense of responsibility for
one's own health, enabled through advancements in the biomedical sphere and
technoscience.

15. Barron H. Lerner, *The Breast Cancer Wars: Hope, Fear, and the Pursuit of
a Cure in Twentieth-Century America* (New York: Oxford University Press, 2003).

16. An array of pins and buttons depicting the sword were utilized by the
WFA and supporters to mark their membership and commitment to the cause.
See Lerner, 43–44.

17. Quoted in Lerner, 43.

18. Many of these posters highlight how the ACS addressed the personal,
specifically the family, as the realm where cancer awareness and vigilance needed
to be cultivated. Through personal responsibility, cancer could be detected and at-
tacked. Cancer is framed here as that which could be met with retaliatory action.

19. Under neoliberal biopolitics, we have witnessed a declining welfare imperative and the increasing absence of the idea of society or of a collective social
good, a heightened individualizing of the administration and management of life,
and a reworking of life beyond its perceived limits. See Melinda Cooper, *Life as
Surplus: Biotechnology and Capitalism in the Neoliberal Era* (Seattle: University of
Washington Press, 2008), 8. Neoliberal biopolitics, as we outline in the introduction to this volume, refers to a range of social, political, and economic rationalities, programs, directives, and policies that work across multiple scales—local,
regional, national, global.

20. For a comprehensive account of breast cancer activism and politics, see
Nadine Ehlers and Shiloh Krupar, eds., "The Body in Breast Cancer," special issue
of *Social Semiotics* 22, no. 1 (2012); Nadine Ehlers, "Risking Safety: Breast Cancer,
Prognosis, and the Strategic Enterprise of Life," *Journal of Medical Humanities*
37, no. 1 (2016): 81–94; and Barbara Ehrenreich, "Welcome to Cancerland: A
Mammogram Leads to a Cult of Pink Kitsch," *Harper's*, November 2001, 43–53.

21. Ehrenreich, "Welcome to Cancerland." David Cantor states that "a new
'biomedical complex' emerged around cancer, characterized by new relationships
between the biological sciences, clinical medicine, the pharmaceutical industry,
and the federal government as a major supporter of research, as well as by a vast

increase in the scale of investment, the numbers of research institutions, and the size of the scientific and medical communities, and all increasingly entangled in emergent Cold War Politics." Refer to Cantor, "Introduction: Cancer Control and Prevention in the Twentieth Century," *Bulletin of the History of Medicine* 81 (2007): 14–15.

22. See, e.g., Samantha King, *Pink Ribbons Inc.: Breast Cancer and the Politics of Philanthropy* (Minneapolis: University of Minnesota Press, 2008). Also refer to Maren Klawiter, *The Biopolitics of Breast Cancer: Changing Cultures of Disease and Activism* (Minneapolis: University of Minnesota Press, 2008), 135–46.

23. This information was available at "Open Letter Concerning the Susan G. Komen Foundation," http://www.discountgunsales.com/SGKF.pdf (accessed November 28, 2014). All reference to the gun has since been removed from the Discount Gun Sales website; however, an archived version of the letter is at http://big.assets.huffingtonpost.com/SGKF.pdf (accessed November 28, 2014).

24. The figure of the pink warrior most often incites white heterosexual women to do this work, because of the technologies/conventions of white heterosexual femininity on which it draws. See Shiloh R. Krupar, "The Biopsic Adventures of Mammary Glam: Breast Cancer Detection and the Promise of Cancer Glamor," *Social Semiotics* 21, no. 5 (2012): 47–82.

25. Krupar, 65; also see Nadine Ehlers and Shiloh Krupar, "Introduction: The Body in Breast Cancer," *Social Semiotics* 21, no. 5 (2012): 1–11.

26. See Clarke et al., *Biomedicalization.*

27. F. M. Hodges, J. S. Svoboda, and R. S. Van Howe, "Prophylactic Interventions on Children: Balancing Human Rights with Public Health," *Journal of Medical Ethics* 28, no. 1 (2002): 10–16, esp. 11.

28. Michel Foucault, "Two Lectures," in *Power/Knowledge: Selected Interviews and Other Writings, 1972–1977*, ed. Colin Gordon, trans. Colin Gordon, Leo Marshall, John Mepham, and Kate Soper (New York: Pantheon Books, 1980), 98.

29. In this operation, groups of individuals are claiming "belonging" to a particular disease or biological classification, representing what Paul Rabinow has called "biosociality"; see Rabinow, "Artificiality and Enlightenment: From Sociobiology to Biosociality," in *Incorporations*, ed. Jonathan Crary and Sanford Kwinter, 234–52 (New York: Zone Books, 1992).

30. See the Hope Band Online Store website, http://cancerhopebands.com/store/index.php?main_page=down_for_maintenance&zenid=7f232407048ee6d67b299217d97be96c (accessed June 28, 2012).

31. See the SeedBallz "Seeds of Hope" product, https://seedballz.com/products/seeds-of-hope-1 (accessed April 28, 2019).

32. Give Hope is an initiative of The Swedish Childhood Cancer Foundation that raises funds to fight against childhood cancer. See http://swedesres.typepad.com/blog/2008/11/give-hope.html (accessed June 28, 2012).

33. Refer to the Miles of Hope Breast Cancer Foundation's website, https:// milesofhope.org/hoops-for-hope-march-16-register-now/ (accessed April 28, 2019).

34. See the Athletes for Cancer website, http://tenacitygames.com/art/ (accessed June 28, 2012).

35. Refer to the Think Before You Pink website, http://thinkbeforeyoupink .org/ (accessed June 28, 2012).

36. See https://hyundaihopeonwheels.org/ (accessed April 28, 2019).

37. See the Susan G. Komen website, http://apps.komen.org/raceforthecure/ (accessed June 28, 2012).

38. Ehrenreich, "Welcome to Cancerland," 51.

39. Amy Lubitow and Mia Davis, "Pastel Injustice: The Corporate Use of Pinkwashing for Profit," *Environmental Justice* 4, no. 2 (2011): 142.

40. See Peggy Orenstein, "Our Feelgood War on Breast Cancer," *New York Times,* April 25, 2013, http://www.nytimes.com/2013/04/28/magazine/our-feel -good-war-on-breast-cancer.html. On the deadly effects of chemotherapy, see the recent study results published in *The Lancet*: Michael Wallington, Emma B. Saxon, Martine Bomb, Rebecca Smittenaar, Matthew Wickenden, Sean McPhail, Jem Rashbass, David Chao, John Dewar, Denis Talbot, Michael Peake, Timothy Perren, Charles Wilson, and David Dodwell, "30-day Mortality after Systemic Anticancer Treatment for Breast and Lung Cancer in England: A Population-Based, Observational Study," *Lancet Oncology* 17 (2016): 1203–16, http://www .thelancet.com/pdfs/journals/lanonc/PIIS1470-2045(16)30383-7.pdf. For earlier U.S.-based findings, see "Chemotherapy Contributes to a Quarter of Cancer Deaths: Study," http://www.abc.net.au/news/2008-11-13/chemotherapy-contrib utes-to-a-quarter-of-cancer/204358 (accessed February 26, 2018).

41. See the Avon Walk website, https://www.avon.com/category/causes/avon -walk (accessed June 28, 2012).

42. Ehrenreich, "Welcome to Cancerland," 52.

43. Dorothy Broom, "Reading Breast Cancer: Reflections on a Dangerous Intersection," *Health* 5, no. 2 (2001): 254.

44. Quoted in Pamela Grossman, "Metastatic Women Are Stranded in a Sea of Pink," *Women's E-news,* November 27, 2012, http://womensenews.org/story /health/121126/metastatic-women-are-stranded-in-the-sea-pink#.UfslyY4kfgR (accessed August 1, 2013).

45. Lauren Berlant, *Cruel Optimism* (Durham, N.C.: Duke University Press, 2011).

46. See the Mission Hope Cancer Center website, http://www.missionhope cancercenter.com/index.html (accessed November 28, 2014).

47. "UAMS Expands Cancer Treatment and Research Facilities," http://www .magnoliareporter.com/news_and_business/regional_news/article_d58c680a -9c30-11df-8230-001cc4c03286.html (accessed November 28, 2014).

48. See the UAMS Winthrop P. Rockefeller Cancer Institute website, http:// www.seed-of-hope.com/ (accessed November 28, 2014).

49. UAMS Winthrop P. Rockefeller Cancer Institute, "About the Seed of Hope," https://cancer.uams.edu/patient-stories/about-the-seeds-of-hope/ (accessed April 28, 2019).

50. Refer to http://www.seed-of-hope.com/about-the-seeds-of-hope/ (accessed November 28, 2014).

51. See the ACS's Hope Lodge website, https://www.cancer.org/treatment /support-programs-and services/patient-lodging/hope-lodge.html (accessed April 28, 2019).

52. "American Cancer Society Raises $22 Million for Hope Lodge Boston Construction," http://www.cancer.org/myacs/NewEngland/AreaHighlights /american-cancer-society-raises-22-million-for-hope-lodge-boston-construction (accessed November 28, 2014). There is also an AstraZeneca Hope Lodge of the American Cancer Society located in the Philadelphia region.

53. On "greenwashing," see Cindi Katz, "Whose Nature, Whose Culture? Private Productions of Space and the 'Preservation' of Nature," in *Remaking Reality: Nature at the Millennium,* ed. Bruce Braun and Noel Castree, 45–62 (London: Routledge, 1998), and Shiloh R. Krupar, *Hot Spotter's Report: Military Fables of Toxic Waste* (Minneapolis: University of Minnesota Press, 2013).

54. Other scholars refer to this as the "U.S. Biomedical TechnoService Complex Inc."; see Clarke et al., *Biomedicalization.*

55. Del Vecchio Good et al., "American Oncology and the Discourse of Hope."

56. Eric Kadish and Stephen G. Post, "Oncology and Hope," *Journal of Clinical Oncology* 13, no. 7 (1995): 1817.

57. Brown, "Shifting Tenses: Reconnecting Regimes of Truth and Hope," 338; see also Kadish and Post, "Oncology and Hope," 1818.

58. Del Vecchio Good et al., "American Oncology and the Discourse of Hope," 75.

59. Del Vecchio Good et al.

60. Brown, "Shifting Tenses–From 'Regimes of Truth' to 'Regimes of Hope,'" 12.

61. Brown, 11.

62. Brown, 11.

63. R. Tate, J. Haritatos, and S. Cole, "HopeLab's Approach to Re-Mission," *International Journal of Learning and Media* 1, no. 1 (2009): 29. See also HopeLab's website, http://www.hopelab.org/ (accessed February 26, 2018).

64. The game's advertising declares that "an epic battle rages deep in the realms of the human body. Colonies of microscopic cancer cells are replicating, attacking, and damaging healthy organs of young people from all across the United States. Enter Roxxi, your courageous and fully-armed nanobot and

medicine's mightiest warrior." See http://www.hopelab.org/innovative-solutions /re-missionTM/ (accessed November 28, 2014).

65. "Re-Mission 2 Video Game Now in Development," http://www.nanopa prika.eu/profiles/blogs/remission-2-video-game-now-in (accessed November 28, 2014).

66. Kate Metropolis, "Steve Cole," Health Games Research, http://www .healthgamesresearch.org/our-publications/featured-colleagues/steve-cole (accessed November 28, 2014).

67. See Onoyemi Benedict, "Medicine's Neglected Spirit: The Positive Therapeutic Effect of Spirituality," on the CTCA's Our Journey of Hope website, https:// www.ourjourneyofhope.com/general-resources?res=35106 (accessed April 28, 2019).

68. The phrase "mother standard of care" seems to imply the ultimate standard of care that, rather than being simply custodial, is representative of love.

69. See, e.g., Robert L. Dupont, "The Healing Power of Faith: Science Explores Medicine's Last Great Frontier," on the CTCA's Our Journey of Hope website, http://www.ourjourneyofhope.com/resources/articles (accessed November 28, 2014). DuPont's review of Harold G. Koenig's book *The Healing Power of Faith: Science Explores Medicine's Last Great Frontier* (New York: Simon and Schuster, 1999) originally appears in *The American Journal of Psychiatry,* August 1, 2001, https://ajp.psychiatryonline.org/doi/full/10.1176/appi.ajp.158.8.1347.

70. Dupont.

71. Dupont.

72. The CTCA's Our Journey of Hope website, "Don't Waste Your Cancer," February 15, 2006, http://ojoh.hopenavigators.com/resources/articles/don-t-waste -your-cancer (accessed November 28, 2014). Excerpts were originally written by John Piper and can now be found in his book *Don't Waste Your Cancer* (Wheaton, Ill.: Crossway, 2011).

73. The CTCA's Our Journey of Hope website, "Atheist Doctors More Likely to Hasten Death: Survey Finds Religious Beliefs Could Affect Care of Terminally Ill Patients," http://www.ourjourneyofhope.com/resources/articles/atheist -doctors-more-likely-to-hasten-death (accessed November 28, 2014). The original article is by Maria Cheng, "Atheist Doctors More Likely to Hasten Death," NBCNews.com, August 26, 2010, http://www.nbcnews.com/id/38866495/ns /health-health_care/t/atheist-doctors-more-likely-hasten-death/.

74. See, e.g., Elizabeth Ward, Ahmedin Jemal, Vilma Cokkinides, Gopal K. Singh, Cheryll Cardinez, Asma Ghafoor, and Michael Thun, "Cancer Disparities by Race/Ethnicity and Socioeconomic Status," *CA: A Cancer Journal for Clinicians* 54, no. 2 (2004): 78–93; Nadine Ehlers, "Breast Cancer," in *Gender: Matter,* ed. Stacy Alaimo, 281–95 (Farmington Hills, Mich.: Macmillan Reference, 2017).

75. National Institutes of Health, National Cancer Institute, "Cancer Health

Disparities," http://www.cancer.gov/about-nci/organization/crchd/cancer-health
-disparities-fact-sheet (accessed July 20, 2016).

76. National Institutes of Health.

77. National Institutes of Health.

78. Designed to increase access to health insurance and high-quality care for
U.S. residents, the ACA's implementation was expected to result in a decrease of
26 million uninsured by 2017. ACA proponents envisioned that greater access to
care and insurance would increase the availability and utilization of preventive
and treatment services, with the goal of improving health outcomes and reducing
health disparities that disproportionately impact minority populations. Refer to
Eileen B. O'Keefe, Jeremy P. Meltzer, and Traci N. Bethea, "Health Disparities and
Cancer: Racial Disparities in Cancer Mortality in the United States, 2000–2010,"
Frontiers in Public Health 3, no. 51 (2015), http://www.ncbi.nlm.nih.gov/pmc
/articles/PMC4398881 (accessed July 20, 2016). At the time of our writing this
chapter (2018), the ACA remains under attack by the Trump administration, and
it's unclear what effects the ACA will have on cancer outcomes and disparities.

79. African Americans incur substantial medical debt compared with whites,
due to health status, income, and insurance disparities. Refer to Nadine Ehlers
and Leslie R. Hinkson, eds., *Subprime Health: Debt, Race, and U.S. Medicine*
(Minneapolis: University of Minnesota Press, 2017); Jacqueline C. Wiltshire,
Keith Elder, Catarina Kiefe, and Jeroan J. Allison, "Medical Debt and Related
Financial Consequences among Older African American Adults," *American Journal of Public Health* 106, no. 6 (2016): 1086–91, http://www.ncbi.nlm.nih.gov
/pubmed/27077346 (accessed July 20, 2016). Moreover, "women are more likely
than men to forgo, delay, and ration medical care because of medical debt"; see
Jacqueline C. Wiltshire, Tyra Dark, R. L. Brown, and Sharina D. Person, "Gender
Differences in Financial Hardships of Medical Debt," *Journal of Health Care for
the Poor and Underserved* 22, no. 1 (2011): 371, http://www.ncbi.nlm.nih.gov
/pubmed/21317529 (accessed July 20, 2016). For a study of medical debt in relation to poverty, health disparities, and the racial divide in homeownership, refer
to Bronwen Lichtenstein and Joe Weber, "Losing Ground: Racial Disparities in
Medical Debt and Home Foreclosure in the Deep South," *Family and Community
Health* 39, no. 3 (2016): 178–87, http://journals.lww.com/familyandcommunity
health/Abstract/2016/07000/Losing_Ground__Racial_Disparities_in_Medical
_Debt.6.aspx (accessed July 20, 2016).

80. S. Lochlann Jain, "Survival Odds: Mortality in Corporate Time," *Current
Anthropology* 52, no. 3 (2011): 46. Also refer to Jain's extensive cultural analysis
and criticism of cancer biocultures in S. Lochlann Jain, *Malignant: How Cancer
Becomes Us* (Berkeley: University of California Press, 2013).

81. "The Beautiful and Bald Movement: Decorating Domes with Love and
Happiness," http://www.beautifulandbald.com/ (accessed November 28, 2014).

82. See "Bald Barbie Campaign Convinces Mattel to Produce New Doll," https://www.redorbit.com/news/health/1112505299/bald-barbie-campaign-con vinces-mattel-to-produce-new-doll/ (accessed April 28, 2019). Also see the "Bald and Beautiful Barbie" Facebook page (last accessed July 11, 2016).

83. Mattel produced a one-off version of the "Hope" Barbie for four-year-old cancer patient Genesis Reyes in early 2011. The company later announced that it would create a bald friend of the Barbie doll for hospital-only circulation. See "Mattel to Make 'Bald Friend of Barbie,'" http://abcnews.go.com/blogs /health/2012/03/29/mattel-to-produce-bald-friend-of-barbie/ (accessed November 28, 2014). "Ella," friend of Barbie, was introduced by Mattel in late 2012 with very limited distribution. A second line was created in 2014. Ella, however, does not reflect the glam possibilities of bald Barbie, and, with her two optional wigs, does more to conform to dominant norms of femininity. See "Mattel Agrees to Produce More Bald Barbie 'Ella' Dolls for Little Kids with Cancer," http://www .huffingtonpost.com.au/entry/mattel-to-continue-bald-ella-doll_n_5548672 (accessed July 11, 2016). On "makeover culture" in relation to cancer, see Shelley Cobb and Susan Starr, "Breast Cancer, Breast Surgery, and the Makeover Metaphor," *Social Semiotics* 22, no. 1 (2012): 83–101; on "glam" as a response to cancer makeover culture, see Krupar, "Biopsic Adventures of Mammary Glam."

84. The original blog post, "Bald Barbie Is an Over-Reach," has been removed from the ACS website. However, a copy of the Becker post is available at the Jack Morton Foundation website, http://thejackmortonfoundation.org/tuesday -january-17-2012/ (accessed November 28, 2014). Becker later apologized for his post in "Bald Barbie Demand Is an Over-Reach–UPDATED," http://acspressroom .wordpress.com/2012/01/13/bald-barbie-demand-is-an-over-reach/ (accessed November 28, 2014).

85. See HCM's website, http://www.hopecancer.org/ (accessed November 28, 2014).

86. Jain, "Survival Odds," 46.

87. See "About The Tutu Project," http://www.thetutuproject.com/about/# .UBXnDI5rr6E (accessed November 28, 2014).

88. Krupar, *Hot Spotter's Report,* 251–69.

89. Michel Foucault, "Questions of Method," in *The Foucault Effect: Studies in Governmentality,* ed. Graham Burchell, Colin Gordon, and Peter Miller (Chicago: University of Chicago Press, 1991), 84. Foucault also states that "I would therefore propose, as a very first definition of critique, this general characterization: the art of not being governed quite so much." See Foucault, "What Is Critique?," in *The Politics of Truth,* ed. Sylvère Lotringer, trans. Lysa Hochroth and Catherine Porter (Los Angeles, Calif.: Semiotext(e), 1997), 45.

90. Foucault, "What Is Critique?," 45.

2. Target

1. W. E. B. Du Bois, *The Philadelphia Negro: A Social Study* (New York: Lippincott, 1899), http://media.pfeiffer.edu/lridener/dss/DuBois/pntoc.html (accessed June 10, 2013).

2. On biological citizenship, see Nikolas Rose, *The Politics of Life: Biomedicine, Power, and Subjectivity in the Twenty-First Century* (Princeton, N.J.: Princeton University Press, 2007), 24–25.

3. Michel Foucault, *Society Must Be Defended: Lectures at the Collège de France 1975–1976*, ed. Mauro Bertani and Alessandro Fontana, trans. David Macey (New York: Picador, 2003), 255; Rose, *Politics of Life*, 24–25. According to Foucault, the fostering of life is fragmented by race or, we could say, racism has been used as a functional mechanism to control the population en masse.

4. Michael Dillon and Andrew W. Neal, *Foucault on Politics, Security and War* (Hampshire, U.K.: Palgrave Macmillan, 2008), 168.

5. This is a modality of governing that administers (in this case) black life via attention to health. Such administration, as Du Bois makes clear and as we go on to show, is not necessarily affirmative.

6. This form of governing began almost immediately after the formal end of slavery. For instance, the Freedman's Bureau and early postslavery law are familiar examples of how black "freedom" was built on constraint. As Katherine Franke has argued, "the containment of African-American liberty within a 'space of regulated freedom' became one of the principal techniques used by the U.S. government to create particularly governable subjects." See Franke, "Not Quite White," http://www.law.columbia.edu/faculty/faculty_writing/facpubs/franke (accessed May 26, 2013). Such governing continues in multiple ways, from the relentless incarceration of black bodies to the racialization of space to the focus of this chapter—inequitable and endangering forms of biomedical administration.

7. Du Bois, *The Philadelphia Negro*, http://media.pfeiffer.edu/lridener/dss/DuBois/pntoc.html. Du Bois explicitly names these social problems as "poverty, ignorance, crime and labor."

8. The irony, here, is that race consciousness within the medical arena is taking place in the very same moment that we see a concerted move toward so-called color-blindness in the broader social sphere. See, e.g., the move away from affirmative action evidenced in the 2007 U.S. Supreme Court case *Parents Involved in Community Schools v. Seattle School District No. 1*, where the Court ruled that it was unconstitutional for school districts to use individualized racial classifications to achieve diversity and/or avoid racial isolation through student assignment.

9. This view is at odds with Rose, who argues that racialized biomedicine is organized around the fostering of life. Refer to Rose, *Politics of Life*, 167.

10. Such knowledge (and practice) is often referred to as anti-blackness. Anti-blackness does not "simply name various forms of violence experienced by Blacks, but the violence that positions sentient beings outside the realm of the Human." James Bliss, "Hope against Hope: Queer Negativity, Black Feminist Theorizing, and Reproduction without Futurity," *Mosaic: A Journal for the Interdisciplinary Study of Literature* 48 (2015): 89. Frank B. Wilderson specifically considers "the meaning of Blackness not—in the first instance—as a variously and unconsciously interpellated identity or as a conscious social actor [animated by legible political interests], but as a structural position of non-communicability in the face of all other positions." Wilderson, *Red, White and Black: Cinema and the Structure of U.S. Antagonisms* (Durham, N.C.: Duke University Press, 2010), 58, emphasis added.

11. Lindon Barrett, *Racial Blackness and the Discontinuity of Western Modernity,* ed. Justin A. Joyce, Dwight A. McBride, and John Carlos Rowe (Urbana: University of Illinois Press, 2014).

12. Alexander G. Weheliye, *Habeas Viscus: Racializing Assemblages, Biopolitics, and Black Feminist Theories of the Human* (Durham, N.C.: Duke University Press, 2014), 19.

13. Within the violent dehumanizing system of U.S. chattel slavery, the black body was medically cared for only as nonhuman property. One example of this can be seen in the experiments of J. Marion Sims, known as the "father of gynecology," who sought to repair the vaginal fistulas of slave women, largely so that their bodies would still be profitable for white owners—in terms of reproductive and other forms of labor. During slavery and beyond, the black body was not only excluded but also called on to service whiteness, that is, to help foster white life. For instance, the practice of grave robbing supported medical experimentation to improve white health—not to support black lives. In fact, through this operation, the bodies of slaves and free blacks were often viewed as worth more dead than alive. Postslavery, the medical arena has been a site in which black subjects have been repeatedly harmed rather than healed. We see this most clearly with the Tuskegee Syphilis Experiments (spanning from 1932 to 1972), which studied the progression of untreated syphilis in African American men who thought they were receiving free health care from the U.S. government; in the appropriation of the Henrietta Lacks cell line (HeLa) to study cancer in the 1950s; and in the disproportionate number of black men diagnosed with schizophrenia in the 1960s due in large part to their connection with civil rights protest activities. De jure and de facto segregation of hospitals, limited access to preventative health care and health insurance, and higher disease burden borne by blacks, among many other examples, show that the biomedical sphere has failed to attend to African American life. *Beyond* the realm of medicine, black citizens have been subjected to dispossession and abandonment through the dismantling of the social wage

(via the destruction of social welfare), through the increasing incarceration of black individuals, and through various practices (such as attacks on public education and affirmative action) that lead or contribute to patterns of cumulative disadvantage. They have also been subjected to various forms of environmental racism—literally existing in what Rinaldo Walcott has called "zones of black death"—in that minority neighborhoods are besieged by hazardous waste sites, industrial pollution, and lead exposure, which in turn creates exponential health risks for poor black populations. See Walcott, "Zones of Black Death: Institutions, Knowledges, and States of Being," 2014 Antipode AAG Lecture, http://antipodefoundation.org/2014/04/02/the-2014-antipode-aag-lecture/ (accessed August 12, 2014); Harriet A. Washington, *Medical Apartheid: The Dark History of Medical Experimentation on Black Americans from Colonial Times to the Present* (New York: Anchor, 2008). Also see Troy Duster, *Backdoor to Eugenics* (New York: Routledge, 2003); Alondra Nelson, *Body and Soul: The Black Panther Party and the Fight against Medical Discrimination* (Minneapolis: University of Minnesota Press, 2011); Dorothy Roberts, *Fatal Invention: How Science, Politics, and Big Business Re-create Race in the Twenty-First Century* (New York: New Press, 2012); and Michelle van Ryn and Steven S. Fu, "Paved with Good Intentions: Do Public Health and Human Service Providers Contribute to Racial/Ethnic Disparities in Health?," *American Journal of Public Health* 93, no. 2 (2003): 248–55. For reports on racial health disparities, refer to Institute of Medicine Report, *Unequal Treatment: Confronting Racial and Ethnic Disparities in Healthcare,* 2002, http://www.iom.edu/Reports/2002/Unequal-Treatment-Confronting-Racial-and-Ethnic-Disparities-in-Health-Care.aspx (accessed May 20, 2012), and the American Medical Association's report *Health Disparities,* http://www.ama-assn.org/resources/doc/mss/ ph_disparities_pres.pdf (accessed May 20, 2012).

14. Du Bois, *The Philadelphia Negro.* Henry A. Giroux refers to this as the "biopolitics of disposability," wherein entire populations are marginalized by race and are socially and environmentally excluded from the attainment of health. Refer to Henry A. Giroux, "Reading Hurricane Katrina: Race, Class, and the Biopolitics of Disposability," *College Literature* 33, no. 3 (2006): 171.

15. Ruth Wilson Gilmore, "Fatal Couplings of Power and Difference: Notes on Racism and Geography," *Professional Geographer* 54, no. 1 (2002): 15–24.

16. See José Esteban Muñoz, "Feeling Brown: Ethnicity and Affect in Ricardo Bracho's *The Sweetest Hangover* (and Other STDs)," *Theatre Journal* 52, no. 1 (2000): 67–79. Here Muñoz argues that we occupy an anti-black and anti-brown normative world and stresses that multiple processes "[block] the Latina/o citizen-subject's trajectory to 'official' citizen-subject political ontology" (68). Unequal access to health is clearly one of these processes, as are the various other forms of medical apartheid to which Latinx are subject. Also see Muñoz, "'Chico, What Does It Feel Like to Be a Problem?': The Transmission of Brownness," in

A Companion to Latino Studies, ed. Juan Flores and Renato Rosaldo, 441–451 (Oxford: Blackwell, 2007).

17. David Theo Goldberg, "Racisms without Racism," *PMLA* 123, no. 5 (2008): 1712–16.

18. See Adele E. Clarke, Janet K. Shim, Laura Mamo, Jennifer Ruth Fosket, and Jennifer R. Fishman, "Biomedicalization: Technoscientific Transformations of Health, Illness, and U.S. Biomedicine," *American Sociological Review* 68, no. 2 (2003): 181–82.

19. Edward J. O'Boyle, "Delivering Health Care in a Financially Broken System," *Personally Speaking,* no. 32 (2007), http://www.mayoresearch.org/files /FINANCIALIZATION32.pdf (accessed May 25, 2013).

20. Stephanie Saul, "FDA Approves a Heart Drug for African-Americans," *New York Times,* June 24, 2005, http://www.nytimes.com/2005/06/24/health /24drugs.html (accessed May 26, 2013).

21. It is important to note here that BiDil is *not* a pharmacogenomic drug. While both the application for the drug's patent and subsequent marketing stressed biological causes for the drug's effectiveness in African Americans, the various clinical studies never tested genes. Instead, as the FDA advisory committee chair Steven E. Nissen stated, "we're using self-identified race as a surrogate for genetic markers." Cited in Roberts, *Fatal Invention,* 178. Race, then, was used as a *proxy* for (supposed) genetic difference.

22. See the Nitromed BiDil homepage, http://www.nitromed.com/pnt/about _bidil.php (accessed May 26, 2013).

23. Jonathon Kahn, "How a Drug Becomes 'Ethnic': Law, Commerce, and the Production of Racial Categories in Medicine," *Yale Journal of Health Policy, Law, and Ethics* 4, no. 1 (2004): Article 1, 11, http://digitalcommons.law.yale.edu /yjhple/vol4/iss1/1 (accessed May 26, 2013).

24. The A-HeFT trial ended early because of the strengths of its results: morbidity was decreased by 43 percent using BiDil, and hospitalization was decreased by 39 percent. It is important to stress here that the trial only enrolled black patients (a total of 1,050 self-identified black patients with class III or IV heart failure). See H. A. Taylor Jr., J. G. Wilson, D. W. Jones, D. F. Sarpong, A. Srinivasan, R. J. Garrison, C. Nelson, and S. B. Wyatt, "Toward Resolution of Cardiovascular Health Disparities in African Americans: Design and Methods of the Jackson Heart Study," *Ethnicity and Disease* 15, no. S6 (2005): 4–17. Also see the BiDil packaging label (of 2005), http://www.accessdata.fda.gov/drugsatfda_docs /label/2005/020727lbl.pdf (accessed May 26, 2013).

25. Jonathon Kahn, *Race in a Bottle: The Story of BiDil and Racialized Medicine in a Post-genomic Age* (New York: Columbia University Press, 2012).

26. George T. H. Ellison, Jay S. Kaufman, Rosemary F. Head, Paul A. Martin, and Jonathon D. Kahn, "Flaws in the U.S. Food and Drug Administration's

Rationale for Supporting the Development and Approval of BiDil as a Treatment for Heart Failure Only in Black Patients," *Journal of Law, Medicine, and Ethics* 36, no. 3 (2008): 449.

27. Jonathon Kahn, "Patenting Race in a Genomic Age," in *Revisiting Race in a Genomic Age*, ed. Barbara A. Koenig, Sandra Soo-Jin Lee, and Sarah S. Richardson (New Brunswick, N.J.: Rutgers University Press, 2008), 135.

28. Roberts argues that "by approving BiDil, only for use in black patients, the FDA emphasized the supposedly distinct—and, it is implied, substandard—quality of black bodies." Roberts, *Fatal Invention,* 176.

29. See, e.g., Susan M. Reverby, "'Special Treatment': BiDil, Tuskegee, and the Logic of Race," *Journal of Law, Ethics, and Medicine* 36, no. 3 (2008): 478–84. She argues, "The evidence appeared to make congestive heart failure seem almost a 'different disease' in 'self-identified' African Americans at the level of population, as 'self-identified' race became the surrogate marker for some other interactive but unknown, biological and environmental process" (480).

30. The FDA approval did link BiDil to genes by highlighting pharmacogenomic information regarding the biomarkers NAT1 and NAT2 for the clinical pharmacology of BiDil, and a substudy of AHeFT—called the Genetic Risk Assessment in Heart Failure (GRAHF) study—also tested the incidence of genotypes related to heart failure. U.S. Department of Health and Human Services, "Isosorbide and Hydralazine," http://www.fda.gov/Drugs/ScienceResearch/Research Areas/Pharmacogenetics/ucm236797.htm. As such, there were attempts to link the supposed racial efficacy of BiDil to genetics. Refer to Jonathan Xavier Inda, *Racial Prescriptions: Pharmaceuticals, Difference, and the Politics of Life* (Surrey, U.K.: Ashgate, 2014), 62–63. Importantly, however, the latest drug label available for BiDil (2005) does not specifically mention genetic or biomarker testing. http://www.accessdata.fda.gov/drugsatfda_docs/label/2005/020727lbl.pdf.

31. It is widely accepted that there are no racial genes, no clear genomic divide between any of society's socially constructed racial categories, and no stable cluster of biomedically relevant genes that is essentially linked with ancestry or skin color.

32. Troy Duster, "Medicine and People of Color: Unlikely Mix—Race, Biology, and Drugs," *San Francisco Chronicle,* March 17, 2003, B7.

33. Pamela Sankar and Jonathon Kahn, "BiDil: Race Medicine or Race Marketing," *Health Affairs* 24 (2005): 457.

34. Inda, *Racial Prescriptions, 77.*

35. For example, in 2004, the fifth annual Multicultural Pharmaceutical Marketing and PR Conference noted, "Major U.S. drug manufacturers are making it a high priority to cultivate relationships with ethnic consumers, physician groups, community networks and other key stakeholder groups to uncover new market growth. . . . Disproportionately high incidence rates of diabetes, obesity, heart

disease, cancer, HIV/AIDS, asthma and other health conditions among these segments require *many strategic and tactical moves* in pharmaceutical marketing and PR." Quoted in Kahn, "How a Drug Becomes 'Ethnic,'" 25, emphasis added.

36. Saul, "FDA Approves a Heart Drug for African-Americans." According to the 2009 Securities and Exchange Commission 10K report filed by NitroMed, the company's sales from BiDil were considerably lower than expected: "$12.1, $15.3, and $14.9 million in 2006, 2007, and 2008, respectively." See Sheldon Krimsky, "The Art of Medicine: The Short Life of a Race Drug," *The Lancet* 379 (2012): 114–15, http://www.councilforresponsiblegenetics.org/page Documents /GRKZJNMMRR.pdf.

37. Kahn, *Race in a Bottle,* 166.

38. Saul, "F.D.A. Approves a Heart Drug for African-Americans."

39. Rose, *Politics of Life,* 25.

40. Rose, 23.

41. Inda argues that genetic researchers take a nonreductive approach to race and genetics, in that they account for the fact that social factors play a role in disease. Social factors, however, are seen simply to trigger "underlying molecular changes in an individual's body." We argue that, in a circular operation, this is reductionist, as it locates disease ultimately in the (racial) body. Inda, *Racial Prescriptions,* 107.

42. Roberts, *Fatal Invention,* 185–87.

43. See Inda, *Racial Prescriptions,* 106, who references our earlier work on this idea.

44. Anne Pollock, *Medicating Race: Heart Disease and Durable Preoccupations with Difference* (Durham, N.C.: Duke University Press, 2012), 165–69; Roberts, *Fatal Invention,* 185–89.

45. Inda, *Racial Prescriptions*; Jonathan Xavier Inda, "Materializing Hope: Racial Pharmaceuticals, Suffering Bodies, and Biological Citizenship," in *Corpus: An Interdisciplinary Reader on Bodies and Knowledge,* ed. Monica J. Casper and Paisley Currah, 61–80 (New York: Palgrave Macmillan, 2011).

46. Pollock, *Medicating Race,* 169.

47. Dylan Ratigan, "Hot-Spotting: It's How, Not How Much," *Huffington Post,* November 28, 2011, http://www.huffingtonpost.com/dylan-ratigan/hotspotting -its-how-not-h_b_1116765.html (accessed November 28, 2011); also J. Hu, F. Wang, J. Sun, R. Sorrentino, and S. Ebadollahi, "A Healthcare Utilization Analysis Framework for Hot Spotting and Contextual Anomaly Detection," in *American Medical Informatics Association Annual Symposium Proceedings,* 2012, 360–69, https://www.ncbi.nlm.nih.gov/pmc/articles/PMC3540544/ (accessed April 29, 2019).

48. The bottom line of U.S. health care reform is cost reduction—the underlying rationale for targeting the costliest 1 percent and coordinating cost-saving

interventions. A 2012 report released by the Agency for Healthcare Research and Quality found that 1 percent of patients accounted for approximately one-fifth of health care spending in the United States in 2009. According to the U.S. Department of Health and Human Services, almost half of total health care spending can be attributed to 5 percent of the population, and the 15 percent most expensive health conditions account for 44 percent of total health care costs. Refer to Bush, "Health Care's Costliest 1%."

49. Planning and zoning laws, development schemes, and rental and mortgage structures were explicitly used to racialize the demographic layout of Camden City in relation to the county. In the 1960s, nearby suburbs and townships used financial and zoning powers to exclusively attract middle- to upper-class white families away from Camden; at the same time, eminent domain was used to remove poor and black residents from those areas. Refer to Howard Gillette Jr., *Camden after the Fall: Decline and Renewal in a Post-industrial City* (Philadelphia: University of Pennsylvania Press, 2006).

50. U.S. Census Bureau, "QuickFacts Beta," http://www.census.gov/quickfacts /table/PST045214/3410000,00.

51. Kareem Fahim, "Rethinking Revitalization; in Crumbling Camden, New Challenges for a Recovery Plan," *New York Times,* November 5, 2006, https:// www.nytimes.com/2006/11/05/nyregion/05camden.html (accessed July 13, 2016); Poverty Research Institute, "Poverty in the City of Camden," April 2007, http://poverty.lsnj.org/Pages/PovertyCityOfCamden041107.pdf (accessed April 29, 2019).

52. U.S. Census Bureau, "QuickFacts Beta." These figures have since shifted. According to 2012–16 estimates, black and "Hispanic or Latino" populations of Camden are roughly equal in number, the medium household income is now $26,214, and individuals living below the poverty line are at 38.4 percent. See https://factfinder.census.gov/faces/nav/jsf/pages/community_facts.xhtml (accessed March 28, 2018).

53. CamConnect, "Camden Facts," 2008, http://www.camconnect.org/data logue/Camden_Facts_08_3-20-08_health.pdf (accessed July 13, 2016).

54. The practice is first attributed to Dr. Jeffrey Brenner. For a popular account of the development of medical hot-spotting, see, e.g., Atul Gawande, "The Hot Spotters," *New Yorker,* January 24, 2011, http://www.newyorker.com /reporting/2011/01/24/110124fa_fact_gawande (accessed November 30, 2012).

55. Bryce Williams, "Medical Hotspotting: When Treating Patients Like Criminals Makes Sense," *Co-Exist* (blog), November 23, 2011, http://www.fast coexist.com/1678856/medical-hotspotting-when-treating-patients-like-crimi nals-makes-sense (accessed May 30, 2013).

56. Peter Bronski, "The Doctor on a Medical Mission," *Vassar: The Alumnae/i Quarterly,* http://vq.vassar.edu/issues/2012/02/pushing-boundaries/the-doctor

-on-a-medical-mission.html (accessed May 30, 2013). Note that the celebratory narrative that has coalesced around Dr. Brenner and the origins of medical hot-spotting in Camden does not address the way that medical data were first gathered in Camden. Nor is it yet clear how medical intelligence is gathered in the expansion of the hot-spotting model elsewhere. Poor residents who reside in medical hot spots may experience the attenuation of their right to privacy in the service of targeted health intervention. The recent project Camden ARISE—"administrative records integrated for service excellence"—raises additional concerns about privacy rights, by integrating data across social services and institutions, including hospitals, jails, and schools. The goal is to locate cross-sector super users and preemptively intervene to contain the costs of not only emergency room visits but also truancy and criminal justice system recidivism."

57. Bush, "Health Care's Costliest 1%."

58. Bronski, "Doctor on a Medical Mission."

59. Aetna Foundation press release, "Aetna Foundation Awards $325,000 in Grants to Train Doctors for 21st-Century Health Care," March 5, 2013, http://news.aetnafoundation.org/ (accessed May 30, 2013).

60. John Blair, "Universal Hot Spotting: The Future of American Medicine in the Face of a Novel Healthcare Delivery Approach," *Triple Helix* (blog), http://asutriplehelix.org/node/185 (accessed May 30, 2013); also see the Frontline video *Doctor Hotspot,* http://video.pbs.org/video/2070853636/ (accessed June 13, 2013).

61. See Atul Gawande, "Seeing Spots," *New Yorker,* January 27, 2011, https://www.newyorker.com/news/news-desk/seeing-spots (accessed May 30, 2013); Gawande, "Hot Spotters." While we have specifically mentioned medical hot-spotting in Camden, New Jersey, there are numerous other pilot programs of patient-focused accountable care occurring across the country, such as the Special Care Program in Seattle for Boeing workers; CareOregon's geomapping of high-cost users as part of its nonprofit health plan that serves Medicare and Medicaid patients; Southcentral Foundation's health care system in Anchorage, Alaska, which targets Alaska Natives to coordinate care and cut costs; and the 2011 launch of the Center for Integrative Medicine, part of the Spectrum Health Medical Group in Grand Rapids, Michigan, which actively seeks out high-frequency patients for treatment of social and medical issues. Basically, the medical hot-spotting program developed in Camden has become a national movement and model (indeed, international). This is evident in the founding of the National Center for Complex Health and Social Needs—spearheaded by the Camden Coalition of Healthcare Providers—to unite groups working on care delivery that targets vulnerable communities in the United States in ways that cost less and improve clinical outcomes. The center was awarded a $1.3 million grant from the Aetna Foundation in 2016. Refer to Lilo H. Stainton, "Camden's

Targeting of Medical 'Hot Spots' Becomes Model for Other Poor Areas," *NJSpotlight*, December 9, 2016, http://www.njspotlight.com/stories/16/12/08/camden-s -targeting-of-medical-hot-spots-becomes-model-for-other-poor-areas/ (accessed July 17, 2018).

62. Michael Omi and Howard Winant, *Racial Formation in the United States* (New York: Routledge, 2015).

63. The institutional racism of medicine includes lack of economic access to health care in relation to racial stratification of the economy; barriers to hospitals and health care institutions due to the closure, relocation, or privatization of hospitals that primarily serve minority populations; inequities in preventive care and treatment based on medical or biological differences, income, and so on; lack of culturally competent care and/or language accessibility; racial disparities in the provision of treatments and inclusion in research; unequal access to emergency care and excessive wait times; deposit requirements as a prerequisite to care; and the refusal of Medicaid patients. For an extended review, refer to Vernellia Randall, "Institutional Racism in U.S. Health Care," Institute on Race, Health Care, and the Law, https://academic.udayton.edu/health/07humanrights /racial01c.htm (accessed April 29, 2019). Another practice of medical redlining that took public notice in California was the requiring of physician "economic credentials" (in addition to professional credentials) to qualify to perform surgeries in a hospital; doctors who serve costly patients could be rejected on the grounds of being "high risk" for financial loss. Robert Weinman, "Medical Red-Lining: 'Economic Credentials' for Physicians," *Clinical Electroencephalography* 27, no. 4 (1996): 6–7. In general, the corporate dominance in U.S. health care has supported increasingly inequitable distribution of health care resources and thus the declining public health conditions of poor and minority urban communities. See David G. Whiteis, "Unhealthy Cities: Corporate Medicine, Community Economic Underdevelopment, and Public Health," *International Journal of Health Services* 27, no. 2 (1997): 227–42, esp. 227.

64. Williams, "Medical Hotspotting." Also see Lisa Duggan, *The Twilight of Equality? Neoliberalism, Cultural Politics, and the Attack on Democracy* (Boston: Beacon Press, 2003); David J. Roberts and Minelle Mahtani, "Neoliberalizing Race, Racing Neoliberalism: Placing 'Race' in Neoliberal Discourses," *Antipode* 42, no. 2 (2010): 248–57; Michael Omi, "'Slippin' into Darkness': The (Re)Biologization of Race," *Journal of Asian American Studies* 13, no. 3 (2010): 343–58.

65. George Lipsitz incisively observes, "Competition for scarce resources in the North American context generates new racial enmities and antagonisms, which in turn promotes new variants of racism." Lipsitz, *American Studies in a Moment of Danger* (Minneapolis: University of Minnesota Press, 2001), 12.

66. In the late 1990s, David G. Whiteis sounded an early warning: "The current emphasis on 'managing' medical care for cost containment disregards the

social and environmental genesis of many health problems." Whiteis, "Unhealthy Cities," 229.

67. The first quotation is by Doug Eby, MD, vice president of medical services for Southcentral Foundation health care system, Anchorage, Alaska, quoted in Bush, "Health Care's Costliest 1%." The second is by Ed Sealover, "'Hot Spotting' May Be Way to Cool Cost of Health Care," *Denver Business Journal*, July 27, 2012, http://www.bizjournals.com/denver/print-edition/2012/07/27/hot-spotting-may -be-way-to-cool-cost.html (accessed June 13, 2013).

68. April Michelle Herndon, "Collateral Damage from Friendly Fire? Race, Nation, Class and the 'War against Obesity,'" *Social Semiotics* 15, no. 2 (2005): 132.

69. Raj Bhopal, "Spectre of Racism in Health and Health Care: Lessons from History and the United States," *BMJ* 316, no. 7149 (1998): 1970–73, http://www .ncbi.nlm.nih.gov/pmc/articles/PMC1113412/ (accessed May 30, 2013).

70. Whiteis, "Unhealthy Cities," 229.

71. William A. Vega, Michael A. Rodriguez, and Elisabeth Gruskin, "Health Disparities in the Latino Population," *Epidemiologic Reviews* 31, no.1 (2009): 99–112.

72. See Michelle Sarche and Paul Spicer, "Poverty and Health Disparities for American Indian and Alaska Native Children: Current Knowledge and Future Prospects," *Annals of the New York Academy of Sciences* 1136 (2008): 126–36.

73. Moon S. Chen, "Cancer Health Disparities among Asian Americans," *Cancer* 104, no. S12 (2005): 2895–2902.

74. See Chandak Ghosh, "Healthy People 2010 and Asian Americans/Pacific Islanders: Defining a Baseline of Information," *American Journal of Public Health* 93, no. 12 (2003): 2093–98; Marguerite J. McNeely and Edward J. Boyko, "Type 2 Diabetes Prevalence in Asian Americans: Results of a National Health Survey," *Diabetes Care* 27, no. 1 (2004): 66–69.

75. Roberts and Mahtani, "Neoliberalizing Race, Racing Neoliberalism," 249, paraphrasing the arguments of David Wilson, *Cities and Race: America's New Black Ghettos* (New York: Routledge, 2006).

76. Neoliberal self-care entails a shift to biological citizenship, from one who possesses rights to services to a manager of individual health risks in a context of enhanced social control and consumer access. Self-care disciplines individuals— targeting individual behaviors—in line with normative models of health, despite any structural issues that might preclude good health. Agency is privatized, as social values are redefined in the terms of market-based interests. Refer to Torin Monahan and Tyler Wall, "Somatic Surveillance: Corporeal Control through Information Networks," *Surveillance and Society* 4, no. 3 (2007): 164; Susanne Bauer, "Societal and Ethical Issues in Human Biomonitoring—A View from Science Studies," *Environmental Health* 7, Suppl. 1 (2008): 1, 8; Henry A. Giroux, "Spectacles of Race and Pedagogies of Denial: Anti-Black Racist Pedagogy under the Reign of Neoliberalism," *Communication Education* 52, no. 3/4 (2003): 209.

77. Dana-Ain Davis, "Narrating the Mute: Racializing and Racism in a Neoliberal Moment," *Souls* 9, no. 4 (2007): 349; Duggan, *The Twilight of Equality*? Our point here is not that all self-care is neoliberal: communities of color and socially/economically disadvantaged groups engage in self-care practices that are not solely determined by neoliberal logics (e.g., radical self-help, undercommons).

78. The neoliberal assertion of race-transcendent agency eclipses the ongoing impacts of structural racism, such as socioeconomic disinvestment in minority neighborhoods and the political neglect of people of color.

79. Bush, "Health Care's Costliest 1%," 32.

80. Frontline, *Doctor Hotspot*.

81. Monahan and Wall, "Somatic Surveillance," 163; Herndon, "Collateral Damage from Friendly Fire?," 132.

82. Loïc Wacquant, "Crafting the Neoliberal State: Workfare, Prisonfare, and Social Insecurity," *Sociological Forum* 25, no. 2 (2010): 218.

83. George L. Kelling and William J. Bratton, "Declining Crime Rates: Insiders' Views of the New York City Story," *Journal of Criminal Law and Criminology* 88, no. 4 (1998): 1217–31; Amy Propen, "Critical GPS: Toward a New Politics of Location," *ACME* 4, no. 1 (2006): 135, https://www.acme-journal.org/index.php/acme/article/view/731.

84. Williams, "Medical Hotspotting."

85. Whether for biosecurity or marketing purposes, spatial profiling sets up the possibility of expectations that can be linked to spaces and populations through the act of targeting. Targeting territorializes such expectations and involves place-particularizing metaphors, masculinist ideas about penetrating and mastering space, and a network logic (i.e., targets are under the purview of a larger, more encompassing gaze and database). Targeting in terms of "seeing-as-destroying" is beyond the scope of this chapter; refer to Derek Gregory, "'In Another Time-Zone, the Bombs Fall Unsafely. . . .': Targets, Civilians and Late Modern War," http://geographicalimaginations.files.wordpress.com/2012/07/gregory-in-another-time-zone_illustrated.pdf (accessed May 30, 2013); Rey Chow, *The Age of the World Target: Self-Referentiality in War, Theory, and Comparative Work* (Durham, N.C.: Duke University Press, 2006); Caren Kaplan, "Precision Targets: GPS and the Militarization of U.S. Consumer Identity," *American Quarterly* 58, no. 3 (2006): 693–713.

86. Jeremy W. Crampton, "The Biopolitical Justification for Geosurveillance," *Geographical Review* 97, no. 3 (2007): 390. Also see Chow, *Age of the World Target*, 40; Kaplan, "Precision Targets," 694–95; and Samuel Weber, *Targets of Opportunity: On the Militarization of Thinking* (New York: Fordham University Press, 2005).

87. Kaplan, "Precision Targets," 697. Medical hot-spotting is dependent on mining for data and the geographical processing of medical metadata—that is, the mass collecting, geographical networking, and commercial deployment of medical data. Set within the historical context of racialized dispossession and biopiracy

in Western medicine, data mining and the metadata-processing industry have the potential to reproduce and amplify racial domination, in terms of both political economy and epistemological politics. In the most general sense, metadata aggregates scale up and interrelate different data sets, providing more material to enhance our understanding of the larger social and environmental genesis of health problems. Yet with medical hot-spotting, the imperative to find high utilizers of the health care system entails a *self-fulfilling process of data analysis*: the sick and disenfranchised are always the population, never the control group, and those who are healthy among the population are statistically illegible, making the population always appear sicker than it might be (note that this part of the critique is directed toward statistical analysis; by no means do we wish to assert that the medically vulnerable and ill are not really very sick). Medical hot-spotting could also be perceived as an auditing practice within a *self-fulfilling political economy.* Just as postindustrial development of infotechnology and "big data" was historically enabled by subverting capital from inner cities and people of color, medical hot-spotting risks contributing to this disinvestment. Medical intelligence and metadata analysis—at the core of medical hot-spotting—essentially represent a new division of labor of the management of the poor and industrial remains; the industry audits the effects and casualties of the process that gave rise to it.

88. Propen, "Critical GPS," 136.

89. Jenna M. Loyd, *Health Rights Are Civil Rights: Peace and Justice Activism in Los Angeles, 1963–1978* (Minneapolis: University of Minnesota Press, 2014), 30; Loïc Wacquant, "From Slavery to Mass Incarceration: Rethinking the 'Race Question' in the US," *New Left Review* 13 (2002): 41–60; Wacquant, "Crafting the Neoliberal State," 197–220.

90. While we are unable to explore this here, medical hot-spotting has been extended into poor white communities. We might see this as part of a broader metaphorical racializing (as nonwhite) those "failed" white citizens who do not live up to ideals of whiteness. See, e.g., Tiffany Willoughby-Herard, *Waste of a White Skin: The Carnegie Corporation and the Racial Logic of White Vulnerability* (Berkeley: University of California Press, 2015).

91. Stephen Graham, *Cities under Siege: The New Military Urbanism* (London: Verso, 2011), 99.

92. Katharyne Mitchell, "Pre-black Futures," *Antipode* 41, no. 1 (2009): 254. Part of the legacy of militarized visual culture, the targeting operations of medical hot-spotting dramatically translate military dreams of high-tech omniscience and rationality into the governance of urban civil society, extending the military–industrial complex into everyday life. See Crampton, "Biopolitical Justification for Geosurveillance"; Graham, *Cities under Siege*, xi; Matthew Sparke, "From Global Dispossession to Local Repossession: Towards a Worldly Cultural Geography of Occupy Activism," in *The New Companion to Cultural Geography,* ed. Huala

Johnson, Richard Schein, and Jamie Winders, 387–408 (Oxford: Wiley-Blackwell, 2013), also available at http://faculty.washington.edu/sparke/ (accessed June 13, 2013).

93. Through the lens of an epistemology of racial Otherness, black subjects could be understood as posing a threat to the health of the population as a whole, in that their ill health (which, as we argue, is produced through past and present social factors) introduces disequilibrium into the population. Rather than addressing the social causes of ill health, however, blacks are in turn blamed as the cause of disequilibrium.

94. Michel Foucault, *The History of Sexuality: Vol 1. An Introduction,* trans. Robert Hurley (Harmondsworth, U.K.: Penguin, 1978), 137.

95. Race may not be biological, but racism, structural disadvantage, and the historical accumulation of suffering undeniably have biological effects that sediment in the black body. In this way, as Anne Pollock notes, race is "fixed enough for action," and simultaneously, as Giroux reminds us, "the color line in America is neither fixed nor static." Pollock, *Medicating Race,* 179; Giroux, "Spectacles of Race," 209.

96. Bliss, "Hope against Hope," 93.

97. See H. Jack Geiger, "The Origins of Community Health Centers," United Health Foundation, n.d., http://optumday.com/UHF/foh_microsite/pdfs/geiger .pdf (accessed April 29, 2019).

98. Nelson, *Body and Soul*; Mary T. Bassett, "Beyond Berets: The Black Panthers as Health Activists," *American Journal of Public Health* 106, no. 10 (2016): 1741–43.

99. Black Panther Party Research Project, "Black Panther Party Platform and Program," http://web.stanford.edu/group/blackpanthers/history.shtml (accessed March 3, 2018).

100. The politics of refusal could also be explored through the important place of health in historical struggles for social change and historical social movements against anti-black violence; see, e.g., Loyd, *Health Rights Are Civil Rights.* On the persistence of the white–black health divide, refer to Nadine Ehlers and Leslie R. Hinkson, eds., *Subprime Health: Debt and Race in U.S. Medicine* (Minneapolis: University of Minnesota Press, 2017).

101. For further examination of the concept of "not yet realized," refer to Judith Butler, interviewed by George Yancy, "What's Wrong with 'All Lives Matter'?," *Opinionator* (blog), January 12, 2015, http://opinionator.blogs.nytimes .com/2015/01/12/whats-wrong-with-all-lives-matter/ (accessed July 13, 2016).

102. National White Coat Die-In demonstrations were held on December 10, 2014.

103. Giroux, "Reading Hurricane Katrina."

104. Renee Lewis, "Medical Students Stage Nationwide Die-In over Racial Bias

in Health Care," Aljazeera America, December 10, 2014, http://america.aljazeera
.com/articles/2014/12/10/medical-studentsferguson.html (accessed July 13,
2016).

105. "Medical Students to Hold Nationwide 'Die-Ins' and Protests Wednesday
Because #BlackLivesMatter," Physicians for a National Health Program, December, 9, 2014, http://www.pnhp.org/news/2014/december/medical-students-to
-hold-nationwide-'die-ins'-and-protests-wednesday-because-blac (accessed July
14, 2016).

106. For example, WhiteCoats4BlackLives is a medical student–run organization that emerged from the National White Coat Die-In demonstrations. To
safeguard the lives and well-being of patients through eliminating racism, members pursue such goals as raising awareness of racism as a public health concern,
ending racial discrimination in medical care, and preparing future physicians to
be advocates for racial justice. The latter involves not only recruiting, hiring, and
retaining minority medical students and physicians but also developing "national
medical school curricular standards that include information about the history
of racism in medicine, unconscious racial bias in medical decision-making, and
strategies for dismantling structural racism." Refer to the organization's website,
http://www.whitecoats4blacklives.org/about (accessed July 13, 2016).

3. Thrive

1. Rachel Colls, "Materialising Bodily Matter: Intra-action and the Embodiment of 'Fat,'" *Geoforum* 38 (2007): 358.

2. Le'a Kent, "Fighting Abjection: Representing Fat Women," in *Bodies out of
Bounds: Fatness and Transgression,* ed. Jana Evans Braziel and Kathleen LeBesco
(Berkeley: University of California Press, 2000), 132.

3. The World Health Organization has established the categories of *overweight* as having a BMI between 25.0 and 29.9 kilograms per square meter and
obesity as having a BMI greater than 30.0 kilograms per square meter. Importantly, obesity scientists and clinicians are presumed to know the "truth" of obesity and to have the moral and intellectual authority to label it a disease and to
prescribe treatment. We could describe such power using Foucault's concept of
the clinical gaze—a panoptic kind of "expert seeing" that determines what will
appear. This gaze shapes the realm of the possible and works to develop hege-
monic norms through which individuals are administered. See World Health
Organization, "Obesity," http://www.who.int/topics/obesity/en/ (accessed October 15, 2013).

4. Susan Bordo, *Unbearable Weight: Feminism, Western Culture, and the
Body* (Berkeley: University of California Press, 1995), 190.

5. Cartesian logic refers to the philosophical and scientific system developed
by René Descartes in the seventeenth century. Descartes viewed the mind as

being wholly separate from (and superior to) the (ideally subservient) corporeal body. This logic structured Enlightenment thought, which continues to undergird Western knowledge systems.

6. *Failure to thrive* (FTT) is a biomedical term used generally in the field of pediatrics. It is defined as "decelerated or arrested physical growth (height and weight measurements fall below the third or fifth percentile, or a downward change in growth across two major growth percentiles) and is associated with abnormal growth and development." See http://www.hopkinsmedicine.org /healthlibrary/conditions/pediatrics/failure_to_thrive_90,P02297/ (accessed December 11, 2016). Within pediatrics, a shift is occurring whereby obesity is variously beginning to be identified as either (1) the "new failure to thrive" or (2) overthriving that must be prevented. On the new failure to thrive, see, e.g., N.S. Harper, "Neglect: Failure to Thrive and Obesity," *Pediatric Clinics of North America* 61, no. 5 (2014): 937–57, http://www.child-encyclopedia.com/child-obesity /according-experts/obesity-prevention-during-infancy-change-focus (accessed April 30, 2019). On overthriving, see http://www.child-encyclopedia.com/child -obesity/according-experts/obesity-prevention-during-infancy-change-focus. In this chapter, we do not address obesity as "overthriving," precisely due to the deadly conditions that produce obesity and the death effects (at times) of obesity itself. This could hardly, in our view, be seen as overthriving. Instead, we take the narrow "obesity as FTT" designation and apply it to individuals and populations more generally. Our central claim is that fat people are seen as failing to thrive and that the counteraffirmation to thrive (through governing interventions that labor to reduce or eradicate weight) works against itself to actually curtail or truncate life.

7. Kent, "Fighting Abjection," 371.

8. Indeed, this is the main motto of one of the key U.S. health care providers/ insurers, Kaiser Permanente. As it says on its primary website, "Nothing matters more than your health. That's why your whole care team is connected—to you, and to each other—to make it faster and easier to get the care you need. From doctors sharing information to improve your care, to digital tools that make it easy to manage your health, everything works together to help you thrive—and fit your life. That's the power of teamwork." See https://thrive.kaiserpermanente .org/ (accessed January 20, 2017).

9. Catherine Waldby, "Stem Cells, Tissue Cultures and the Production of Biovalue," *Health* 6, no. 3 (2002): 310.

10. Nikolas Rose, *The Politics of Life Itself: Biomedicine, Power, and Subjectivity in the Twenty-First Century* (Princeton, N.J.: Princeton University Press, 2007), 32.

11. Exploring this delineation is beyond the scope of this chapter. It is, however, a necessary area for further investigation.

12. World Health Organization Fact Sheet, "Obesity and Overweight," http://

www.who.int/en/news-room/fact-sheets/detail/obesity-and-overweight (accessed May 2, 2019).

13. For adult obesity rates, see Centers for Disease Control and Prevention, "Adult Obesity Facts," https://www.cdc.gov/obesity/data/adult.html (accessed May 1, 2019). For child obesity rates, see Centers for Disease Control and Prevention, "Childhood Obesity Facts," https://www.cdc.gov/obesity/data/childhood.html (accessed May 1, 2019).

14. See U.S. Department of Health and Human Services, "Overweight and Obese Statistics," https://www.niddk.nih.gov/health-information/health-statistics/Pages/overweight-obesity-statistics.aspx (accessed January 7, 2016).

15. U.S. Department of Health and Human Services.

16. For a discussion and problematization of the concept of "excess deaths" related to obesity, see Julie Guthman, "Fatuous Measures: The Artificial Construction of the Obesity Epidemic," *Critical Public Health* 23, no. 3 (2013): 263–73.

17. Fitness, here, signified whether one was a worthy American or not, a point we return to later.

18. Associated Press, "Obesity Bigger Threat Than Terrorism?," March 1, 2006. For more about bioterrorism, "fatwa(r)" rhetoric, and an analysis of the "war against obesity," refer to April Michelle Herndon, "Collateral Damage from Friendly Fire? Race, Nation, Class and the 'War against Obesity,'" *Social Semiotics* 15, no. 2 (2005): 128–41. Also see Charlotte Biltekoff, "The Terror Within: Obesity in Post 9/11 U.S. Life," *American Studies* 48, no. 3 (2007): 29–48.

19. American Medical Association, "AMA Adopts New Policies on Second Day of Voting at Annual Meeting," 2013, https://ama-assn.org/ (accessed June 25, 2013), emphasis added. Also see http://www.theatlantic.com/health/archive/2015/03/how-obesity-became-a-disease/388300/.

20. Shiriki Kumanyika and Ross Brownson, *Handbook of Obesity Prevention: A Resource for Health Professionals* (New York: Springer, 2007). Also see Trust for America's Health and Robert Wood Johnson Foundation, "State of Obesity," fact sheet, http://stateofobesity.org/healthcare-costs-obesity/ (accessed January 11, 2017).

21. Kathryn Pauly Morgan, "Foucault, Ugly Ducklings, and Technoswans: Analyzing Fat Hatred, Weight-loss Surgery, and Compulsory Biomedicalized Aesthetics in America," *International Journal of Feminist Approaches to Bioethics* 4, no. 1 (2011): 204.

22. "Governing Obese Bodies in a Control Society," *Junctures: The Journal for Thematic Dialogue* 11 (2008), http://www.junctures.org/index.php/junctures/article/view/35/372.

23. Morgan, "Foucault, Ugly Ducklings, and Technoswans," 197.

24. On the critique of BMI scales, see, e.g., Bethan Evans and Rachel Colls, "Measuring Fatness, Governing Bodies: The Spatialities of the Body Mass Index (BMI) in Anti-obesity Politics," *Antipode* 41 (2009): 1051–83.

25. See U.S. Department of Health and Human Services, NIH, "Overweight and Obese Statistics," https://www.niddk.nih.gov/health-information/health-sta tistics/Pages/overweight-obesity-statistics.aspx (accessed December 11, 2016), emphasis added. They do conclude with the following: "Many factors can lead to energy imbalance and weight gain. They include genes, eating habits, how and where people live, attitudes and emotions, life habits, and income." However, personal eating habits—"calories in"—are clearly presented as the primary cause of obesity, as the emphasized portion of the quote demonstrates.

26. Nicole L. Novak and Kelly David Brownell, "Obesity: A Public Health Approach," *Psychiatry Clinics of North America* 34, no. 4 (2011): 895–909.

27. For discussion of the Alexander Draper case, see Shauneen M. Garrahan and Andrew W. Eichner, "Tipping the Scale: A Place for Childhood Obesity in the Evolving Legal Framework of Child Abuse and Neglect," *Yale Journal of Health Policy, Law, and Ethics* 12, no. 2 (2012): 336–70. For discussion of the Anamarie Regino case, see Herndon, "Collateral Damage from Friendly Fire?"

28. *The U.S. Weight Loss and Diet Control Market*, 15th ed. (Marketdata LLC, 2019), https://www.giiresearch.com/report/md191871-us-weight-loss-diet -control-market-11th-edition.html (accessed May 2, 2019).

29. Lauren Berlant, "Risky Bigness: On Obesity, Eating, and the Ambiguity of 'Health,'" in *Against Health: How Health Became the New Morality,* ed. Jonathan M. Metzl and Anna Kirkland (New York: New York University Press, 2010), 31.

30. Michel Foucault, *Society Must Be Defended: Lectures at the Collège de France 1975–1976,* trans. David Macey (New York: Picador, 2003), 139.

31. See https://www.rxlist.com/alli-side-effects-drug-center.htm (accessed April 30, 2019).

32. Tetsuji Takayama, Shinichi Katsuki, Yasuo Takahashi, Motoh Ohi, Shuichi Nojiri, Sumio Sakamaki, Junji Kato, Katsuhisa Kogawa, Hirotsugu Miyake, and Yoshiro Niitsu, "Aberrant Crypt Foci of the Colon as Precursors of Adenoma and Cancer," *New England Journal of Medicine* 339, no. 18 (1998): 1277–84.

33. Morgan, "Foucault, Ugly Ducklings, and Technoswans," 194.

34. Walter J. Pories, "Bariatric Surgery: Risks and Rewards," *Journal of Clinical Endocrinology and Metabolism* 93, no. 11 (2008): S89–96, http://press.endo crine.org/doi/full/10.1210/jc.2008-1641#sthash.6ishn6PU.dpuf. See also Su Hsin Chang, Carolyn R. T. Stoll, Jihyun Song, J. Esteban Varela, Christopher J. Eagon, and Graham A. Colditz, "Bariatric Surgery: An Updated Systematic Review and Meta-analysis, 2003–2012," *JAMA Surgery,* 149, no. 3 (2014): 275–87.

35. See the Centers for Disease Control and Prevention website, http://www .cdc.gov/ncbddd/disabilityandhealth/obesity.html (accessed January 20, 2017).

36. See Morgan Downey and Christopher D. Still, "The Affordable Care Act's Impact on Persons with Obesity," http://www.downeyobesityreport.com/wp -content/uploads/The-Affordable-Care-Act2.pdf (accessed December 1, 2016). See also http://www.reuters.com/article/us-obesity-idUSBRE83T0C820120430.

37. White House Task Force on Childhood Obesity, *Solving the Problem of Childhood Obesity within a Generation* (Washington, D.C.: Executive Office of the President of the United States, 2010).

38. White House, 23, emphasis added. Importantly, pillar 3, "Providing Healthy Food in Schools," and pillar 4, "Access to Healthy, Affordable Food," do address wider societal factors outside individual behavior. In relation to pillar 4, the report specifically recommends the following: "increase physical access to healthy food by eliminating food deserts (primarily through the Healthy Food Financing Initiative); increase the production of fruits, vegetables and whole grains; evaluate the effect of subsidies and sales taxes; encourage the food and restaurant industry to develop healthy foods for young people; and address links of hunger and obesity by increasing participation rates in USDA nutrition assistance programs (such as school lunches and SNAP—commonly known as food stamps)." These recommendations reflect the changes many antiracist, antipoverty, and antihunger activists have long been advocating for. Of note, however, is that they follow recommendations that give priority to individual action, and their implementation is a long way in coming. For further analysis of the report, particularly its racial and gendered dimensions, see Jeanne Firth, "Healthy Choices and Heavy Burdens: Race, Citizenship and Gender in the 'Obesity Epidemic,'" *Journal of International Women's Studies* 13, no. 2 (2012): 33–50. These efforts are under review in the Trump administration.

39. Julie Guthman and Melanie DuPuis, "Embodying Neoliberalism: Economy, Culture, and the Politics of Fat," *Environment and Planning D: Society and Space* 24 (2006): 427–48, esp. 229.

40. Guthman and DuPuis, 443.

41. See https://www.niddk.nih.gov/health-information/health-statistics/Pages/overweight-obesity-statistics.aspx (accessed January 20, 2017).

42. Researchers measure food deserts in various ways. However, when they label an area a "food desert," they tend to mean that those individuals (and the community as a whole) living within the area lack easy access to healthy food.

43. Refer to "Unshared Bounty: How Structural Racism Contributes to the Creation and Persistence of Food Deserts," http://www.racialjusticeproject.com/wp-content/uploads/sites/30/2012/06/NYLS-Food-Deserts-Report.pdf, quote on 6. Note that the USDA's Economic Research Service found that "in all but very dense urban areas, the higher the percentage of minority population, the more likely the area is to be a food desert." See Paula Dutko, Michele Ver Ploeg, and Tracey Farrigan, "Characteristics and Influential Factors of Food Deserts," https://www.ers.usda.gov/webdocs/publications/45014/30940_err140.pdf (accessed April 30, 2019).

44. As many food and antipoverty activists have noted, there is a correlation between hunger and fatness. According to the Center on Hunger and Poverty,

lack of resources can lead to weight gain because (1) individuals might maximize caloric intake with inexpensive high-calorie food, (2) individuals might choose food quantity—to abate hunger—over food quality, (3) individuals might overeat when food is available, to ward against times when it will be scarce, and (4) the body might adapt physiologically to store fat to compensate for times when food is scarce. See "The Paradox of Hunger and Obesity in America," http://www.agnt .org/humane/hungerandobesity.pdf (accessed January 11, 2017).

45. Julie Guthman, "Doing Justice to Bodies? Reflections on Food Justice, Race, and Biology," *Antipode* 46, no. 4 (2014): 1153–71, esp. 1165.

46. Didier Fassin, "Another Politics of Life Is Possible," *Theory, Culture, and Society* 26, no. 5 (2009): 44–60. On subcitizenship, see Matthew Sparke, "Austerity and the Embodiment of Neoliberalism as Ill-Health: Towards a Theory of Biological Sub-citizenship," *Social Science and Medicine* 187 (2017): 287–95. He argues, "The 'sub' in sub-citizenship is used . . . to elucidate power relations and processes of subordination that simple binary accounts of citizenship and its others tend to foreclose. Instead, attention to the power relations and processes producing *sub*-citizenship opens up questions about differential degrees and dynamics of health rights disenfranchisement, their various incarnations in adverse incorporation as well as exclusion, and their uneven impacts on actual health outcomes."

47. Lauren Berlant, *Cruel Optimism* (Durham, N.C.: Duke University Press, 2011).

48. See Julie Guthman, "Binging and Purging: Agrofood Capitalism and the Body as Socioecological Fix," *Environment and Planning A* 47 (2015): 2531.

49. Natalie Boero, "Bypassing Blame: Bariatric Surgery and the Case of Biomedical Failure," in *Biomedicalization: Technoscience, Health, and Illness in the U.S.,* ed. Adele. E. Clarke, Laura Mamo, Jennifer Ruth Fosket, Jennifer R. Fishman, and Janet K. Shim (Durham, N.C.: Duke University Press, 2010), 315.

50. Foucault, *Society Must Be Defended,* 258.

51. Catherine Waldby and Robert Mitchell, *Tissue Economies: Blood, Organs, and Cell Lines in Late Capitalism* (Durham, N.C.: Duke University Press, 2006), 115.

52. Daniel Del Vecchio and Hetal Fichadia, "Autologous Fat Transplantation—A Paradigm Shift in Breast Reconstruction," in *Breast Reconstruction: Current Techniques,* ed. Marzia Salgarello (IntechOpen, 2012), http://www.intech open.com/books/breast-reconstruction-current-techniques (accessed March 11, 2012).

53. See Sharon Begley, "All Natural: Why Breasts Are the Key to the Future of Regenerative Medicine," *Wired,* November 2010, https://www.wired .com/2010/10/ff-futureofbreasts/; P. Zuk, "Adipose-Derived Stem Cells in Tissue Regeneration: A Review," *ISRN Stem Cells* (2013): 1–35.

54. Begley, "All Natural."

55. Cited in Scott Terranella, "Fat: Source of Stem Cells: Researchers Report Turning Fat Cells into Muscle," ABC News, April 10, [no year], http://abcnews .go.com/Health/story?id=117521 (accessed March 11, 2014).

56. Bruce Carlson, *Principles of Regenerative Biology* (Burlington, Mass.: Academic Press, 2007), 244.

57. NIH, U.S. National Library of Medicine, https://clinicaltrials.gov/ct2/res ults?cond=&term=adipose+stem+cells&cntry=&state=&city=&dist. This figure is current as of April 2019.

58. Jeffery M. Gimble, Adam J. Katz, and Bruce A. Bunnell, "Adipose-Derived Stem Cells for Regenerative Medicine," *Circulation Research: Journal of the American Heart Association* 100 (2007): 1249.

59. See Zuk, "Adipose-Derived Stem Cells in Tissue Regeneration." The clinical potential of human ADSCs is still unclear and requires deeper investigation. See Michelle Locke, Vaughan Feisst, and P. Rod Dunbar, "Concise Review: Human Adipose-Derived Stem Cells: Separating Promise from Clinical Need," *Stem Cells* 29, no. 3 (2011): 404–11.

60. Begley, "All Natural."

61. In saying this, we are suggesting that breasts are not necessary for the subject to stay alive. Undeniably, however, breasts play a large role in reproductive labor (that is, in terms of breast-feeding) and thus in the survival of children.

62. See "New Breast Reconstruction Procedure Demonstrates Long Term Success in European Trial; Data Reported from Cytori's RESTORE-2 Study of the Celution(R) System," http://ir.cytori.com/files/doc_news/CYTX_News _2011_3_2_General.pdf. Two clinical trials have been conducted using RE-STORE, and it has been approved for use (and is being used) in Australia. http:// ir.cytori.com/investor-relations/News/news-details/2013/Cytoris-Celution-Sys tem-Approved-in-Australia-for-Processing-and-Delivering-Adipose-Derived -Regenerative-Cells/default.aspx.

63. Ramon Pérez-Cano, J. J. Vranckx, J. M. Lasso, C. Calabrese, B. Merck, A. M. Milstein, E. Sassoon, E. Delay, and E. M. Weiler-Mithoff, "Prospective Trial of Adipose-Derived Regenerative Cell (ADRC)-Enriched Fat Grafting for Partial Mastectomy Defects: The RESTORE-2 Trial," *European Journal of Surgical Oncology* 38, no. 5 (2012): 382–89.

64. See the Neopec homepage, http://www.neopec.com.au/.

65. The clinical trial for the Neopec technology was completed in late 2012, and proof of principle was established. See "Neopec Clinical Trial Completed," http://www.neopec.com.au/index.php/recent-news/89–2012/132-neopec-clinical -trial-completed (accessed January 20, 2017).

66. See "Stem Cell Therapy: How American CryoStem Is Leading the Way in Preparing Individuals for Personalized Regenerative Medicine," https://www

.prnewschannel.com/2016/07/14/stem-cell-therapy-how-american-cryostem-is-leading-the-way-in-preparing-individuals-for-personalized-regenerative-medicine/ (accessed January 11, 2017).

67. Melinda Cooper, *Life as Surplus: Biotechnology and Capitalism in the Neoliberal Era* (Seattle: University of Washington Press, 2008), 125.

68. Morikuni Tobita, "Adipose-Derived Stem Cells: Current Findings and Future Perspectives," *Discovery Medicine* 11, no. 57 (2011): 160–70. Tobita argues, however, that the effect of ADSCs is a controversial topic: other studies have reported that ADSCs inhibited breast cancer metastasis. Regardless, as he notes, the effects of adipose tissue on tumor cells should be carefully examined before future applications of stem cells therapies.

69. Waldy and Mitchell, *Tissue Economies,* 56.

70. Rose, *Politics of Life Itself,* 25.

71. Rose, 25.

72. See http://fattransfernewyork.com/cryopreservation-adult-stem-cells/ (accessed January 6, 2016).

73. Waldby and Mitchell, *Tissue Economies,* 83.

74. BioLife Cell Bank is now closed. Their "Banking Packages" website had previously been available at: http://www.biolifecellbank.com/for-patients/service-packages/.

75. Refer to "Stem Cell 'Cowboy Culture' Emerging in Texas—and Australia" in the Stem Cell Foundation of Australia e-newsletter, April 2013, http://www.stemcellfoundation.net.au/news/newsletters/april-2013. Also see Sophie Scoot and Alison Branley, "Stem Cell Warning: Experts Fear Experimental Treatments Will Lead to Serious Injury," ABC News, December 13, 2013, http://www.abc.net.au/news/2013-12-18/stem-cell-warning3a-experts-fear-experimental-treatments-will-/5164636.

76. For instance, see Gina Kolata, "A Cautionary Tale of 'Stem Cell Tourism,'" *New York Times,* June 22, 2016, https://www.nytimes.com/2016/06/23/health/a-cautionary-tale-of-stem-cell-tourism.html (accessed June 20, 2016).

77. American Cancer Society, "Cancer Facts and Figures, 2017–2018," https://www.cancer.org/content/dam/cancer-org/research/cancer-facts-and-statistics/breast-cancer-facts-and-figures/breast-cancer-facts-and-figures-2017-2018.pdf. (accessed July 23, 2018). "Crude 10-year survival rates are 80% for white women, 78% for Hispanic American women, 66% for black women, and 82% for Asian women." See Javaid Iqbal, Ophira Ginsburg, and Paula A. Rochon, "Differences in Breast Cancer Stage at Diagnosis and Cancer-Specific Survival by Race and Ethnicity in the United States," *JAMA* 313, no. 2 (2015): 166.

78. American Cancer Society, "Cancer Facts and Figures for African Americans, 2016–2018," http://www.cancer.org/acs/groups/content/@editorial/documents/document/acspc-047403.pdf (accessed July 24, 2018).

79. Joseph H. Shin, "Socioeconomic Disparities in Immediate Breast Reconstruction: Public vs. Private Insurance," American Association of Plastic Surgeons Annual Conference, 2013, http://meeting.aaps1921.org/abstracts/2013/19.cgi.

80. Just over a decade ago, the average cost of TRAM flap reconstructions was at $19,607 (range, $11,948–$49,402), compared with $15,497 for prosthetic reconstructions (range, $6,422–$40,015). See Scott Spear, Samir Mardini, and Jason C. Ganz, "Resource Cost Comparison of Implant-Based Breast Reconstruction versus TRAM Flap Breast Reconstruction," *Plastic and Reconstructive Surgery* 112, no. 1 (2003): 101–5. According to *US News,* the cost of breast reconstruction has more than tripled in the last decade. Refer to Kathleen Doheny, "Few Women Get Breast Reconstruction after Mastectomy," *US News,* December 8, 2011, http://health.usnews.com/health-news/family-health/cancer/articles/2011/12/08/few-women-get-breast-reconstruction-after-mastectomy-study.

81. As Rose has remarked, individuals are increasingly expected to partake of the ethic of active citizenship: "This is an ethic in which the maximization of lifestyle, potential, health, and quality of life has become almost obligatory, and where negative judgments are directed toward those who will not [or cannot], for whatever reason, adopt an active, informed, positive, and prudent relation to the future." Rose, *Politics of Life Itself,* 25.

82. Kathleen LeBesco, "Neoliberalism, Public Health, and the Moral Perils of Fatness," *Critical Public Health* 21, no. 2 (2011): 161.

83. See http://haescommunity.com/.

84. This campaign has not been without its critics. In an open letter, the organization NoLose critiqued the I STAND images as being an example of white fat activism that failed to address the socioeconomic and race-based specificities of fat politics or represent the voices of people of color and poor communities. See http://nolose.org/about/policy/fat-white-activism-poc/ (accessed July 24, 2018).

85. Berlant, *Cruel Optimism,* 115.

86. Berlant, 115.

87. Emily Yates-Doerr and Megan A. Carney, "Demedicalizing Health: The Kitchen as a Site of Care," *Medical Anthropology* 35, no. 4 (2016): 313.

88. Gimble et al., "Adipose-Derived Stem Cells for Regenerative Medicine," 1249. In this incantation, fat banking is ostensibly imagined—albeit perhaps problematically—as a solution to the obesity epidemic. This has the potential to rework existing discourses of obesity, though the reality of such practices is still a long way off, and the ethics is questionable.

4. Secure

1. Mark Mather, Linda A. Jacobsen, and Kelvin M. Pollard, "Aging in the United States," *Population Bulletin* 70, no. 2 (2015), http://www.prb.org/pdf16/aging-us-population-bulletin.pdf (accessed March 5, 2018).

2. Michel Foucault, *Society Must Be Defended: Lectures at the Collège de France 1975–1976*, trans. David Macey (New York: Picador, 2003), 244.

3. Melinda Cooper, "Resuscitations: Stem Cells and the Crisis of Old Age," *Body and Society* 12, no. 1 (2006): 2.

4. Cooper, 14.

5. Recall, as we outline in the introduction to this volume, that biopolitics is generally a politics of security—securing the population against anything from endemic diseases to criminal conduct, particularly through the biologized apparatuses of health and medicine.

6. *Biocultures of aging* refers to various cultural spheres where biomedical attitudes toward age pervade how we think about age and the process of aging.

7. Peter Laslett, *A Fresh Map of Life: The Emergence of the Third Age* (London: Weidenfeld and Nicolson, 1989).

8. For a range of definitions of successful aging, see Ann Bowling, "Aspirations for Older Age in the 21st Century: What Is Successful Aging?," *International Journal of Aging and Human Development* 64, no. 3 (2007): 263–97.

9. Julia Rozanova, "Discourse of Successful Aging in *The Globe & Mail*: Insights from Critical Gerontology," *Journal of Aging Studies* 24, no. 4 (2010): 215.

10. Paul Higgs, Miranda Leontowitsch, Fiona Stevenson, and Ian Rees Jones, "Not Just Old and Sick: The 'Will to Health' in Later Life," *Aging and Society* 29 (2009): 690.

11. Cooper, "Resuscitations," 5.

12. Brett Neilson, "Anti-ageing Cultures, Biopolitics and Globalisation," *Cultural Studies Review* 12, no. 2 (2006): 149–64.

13. Some topics not covered here include annuities, pensions, and life insurance to anti-aging products to Medicare policy.

14. This is particularly the case in the American context, where individualism continues to be highly prized.

15. Neena L. Chappell, Ellen Gee, Lynn McDonald, and Michael Stones, *Aging in Contemporary Canada* (Toronto: Prentice-Hall, 2002), 12; Stephen Katz and Barbara L. Marshall, "Is the Functional 'Normal'? Aging, Sexuality and the Bio-marking of Successful Living," *History of the Human Sciences* 17, no. 1 (2004): 63.

16. Sharon R. Kaufman, "Making Longevity in an Aging Society: Linking Ethical Sensibility and Medicare Spending," *Medical Anthropology* 28, no. 4 (2009): 317.

17. Stephen Katz and Barbara Marshall, "New Sex for Old: Lifestyle, Consumerism, and the Ethics of Aging Well," *Journal of Aging Studies* 17 (2003): 12.

18. Courtney Everts Mykytyn, "Anti-aging Is Not Necessarily Anti-death: Bioethics and the Front Lines of Practice," *Medicine Studies* 1 (2009): 214.

19. "Resources for Encore Seekers," http://encore.org/resources/encore-seekers/ (accessed January 23, 2018).

20. "Energize Your Community with Experience," http://www.reserveinc
.org/ (accessed January 23, 2018); "Become a ReServist," http://www.reserveinc
.org/become-a-reservist (accessed January 23, 2018).

21. John Wallis Rowe and Robert L. Kahn, *Successful Aging* (New York: Random House, 1998).

22. Stephen Katz, "Busy Bodies: Activity, Aging, and the Management of Everyday Life," *Journal of Aging Studies* 14, no. 2 (2000): 142.

23. The geographies of seniors and eldercare entail various forms of migration, medical tourism, and segmented landscapes of retirement communities. Refer to Stephen Katz, "Old Age as Lifestyle in an Active Society," Doreen B. Townsend Center Occasional Paper 19 (1999); Kevin McHugh, "The 'Ageless Self'? Emplacement of Identities in Sun Belt Retirement Communities," *Journal of Aging Studies* 14, no. 1 (2000): 103–15.

24. The Milken Institute—the think tank behind the ranking—cites AARP (formerly the American Association of Retired Persons) and National Aging in Place Council research that up to 90 percent of older people want to age in place and at home to maintain their independence. Refer to Milken Institute, "Best Cities of Successful Aging," 2014, http://successfulaging.milkeninstitute.org/2014 /best-cities-for-successful-aging-report-2014.pdf (accessed January 23, 2018); National Aging in Place Council, "Act III: Your Plan for Aging in Place," http:// www.ageinplace.org/ (accessed January 23, 2018).

25. Isabel Dyck, Pia Kontos, Jan Angus, and Patricia McKeever, "The Home as a Site for Long-Term Care: Meanings and Management of Bodies and Spaces," *Health and Place* 11 (2005): 173–85; Qin Ni, Ana Belén García Hernando, and Paul de la Cruz, "The Elderly's Independent Living in Smart Homes: A Characterization of Activities and Sensing Infrastructure Survey to Facilitate Services Development," *Sensors* 15 (2015): 11312–62; Maggie Mort, Celia Roberts, and Blanca Callén, "Ageing with Telecare: Care or Coercion in Austerity?," *Sociology of Health and Illness* 35, no. 6 (2013): 799–812; N. M. Barnes, N. H. Edwards, D. A. D. Rose, and P. Garner, "Lifestyle Monitoring—Technology for Supported Independence," *Computing and Control Engineering Journal,* August 1998, 169–74.

26. Ilkka Korhonen, Juha Pärkkä, and Mark Van Gils, "Health Monitoring in the Home of the Future," *IEEE Engineering in Biology and Medicine Magazine,* May/June 2003, 66–73.

27. Kimberly Leonard and Josh Israel, "Telehealth Bill Aims to Expand Health IT Access for Home Care Providers," Center for Public Integrity, March 22, 2011, https://www.publicintegrity.org/2011/03/22/3688/telehealth-bill-aims -expand-health-it-access-home-care-providers (accessed January 23, 2018).

28. Stealth Health, http://stealthhealth.co/ (accessed January 23, 2018).

29. Reminder Rosie, http://www.reminder-rosie.com/ (accessed January 23, 2018).

30. The Pill Pets are brightly colored, cuddly toys made of silicon with com-

puterized screens that display instructions on taking medication. For the Pill Pets to thrive, their reminders to take medication must be followed; if they are not paid attention, the Pill Pets will become ill and eventually die. Refer to AgeLab, "Pharm Animals and Pill Pets," http://agelab.mit.edu/pharm-animals-pill-pets (accessed January 23, 2018).

31. Refer to http://www.gerijoy.com/ (accessed March 19, 2018).

32. Neilson, "Anti-ageing Cultures, Biopolitics and Globalisation," 12.

33. Carolyn Cartier, "From Home to Hospital and Back Again: Economic Restructuring, End of Life, and the Gendered Problems of Place-Switching Health Services," *Social Science and Medicine* 56 (2003): 2289–2301; Joan Liaschenko, "The Moral Geography of Home Care," *Advances in Nursing Science* 17, no. 2 (1994): 16–26; Lauren Penney, "The Uncertain Bodies and Spaces of Aging in Place," *Anthropology and Aging Quarterly* 34, no. 3 (2013): 113–25.

34. Katz and Marshall, "New Sex for Old," 12. See also Martha Albertson Fineman, "'Elderly' as Vulnerable: Rethinking the Nature of Individual and Societal Responsibility," Emory Legal Studies Research Paper No. 12-224, June 20, 2012, http://dx.doi.org/10.2139/ssrn.2088159 (accessed January 23, 2018).

35. Martha B. Holstein and Meredith Minkler, "Self, Society, and the 'New Gerontology,'" *Gerontologist* 43, no. 6 (2003): 788; Katz and Marshall, "Is the Functional 'Normal'?"

36. David J. Ekerdt, "The Busy Ethic: Moral Continuity between Work and Retirement," *Gerontologist* 26, no. 3 (1986): 239–44.

37. Mykytyn, "Anti-aging Is Not Necessarily Anti-death," 218–19.

38. Mykytyn, 216.

39. Katz and Marshall, "Is the Functional 'Normal'?," 63.

40. Katz and Marshall, 68–69.

41. Katz and Marshall, 63.

42. Katz and Marshall, 58.

43. Holstein and Minkler, "Self, Society, and the 'New Gerontology,'" 792, citing Sarah Harper, "Constructing Later Life/Constructing the Body: Some Thoughts from Feminist Theory," in *Critical Approaches to Ageing and Later Life*, ed. Anne Jamieson, Sarah Harper, and Christina R. Victor (Buckingham, U.K.: Open University Press, 1997), 167.

44. Holstein and Minkler, "Self, Society, and the 'New Gerontology,'" 787.

45. Refer to Fitbit, https://www.fitbit.com/home (accessed January 23, 2018); Oura, https://ouraring.com/ (accessed January 23, 2018).

46. Courtney Everts Mykytyn, "A History of the Future: Emergence of Contemporary Anti-ageing Medicine," *Sociology of Health and Illness* 23, no. 2 (2010): 185.

47. Nicholas Rose, *The Politics of Life Itself, Biomedicine, Power, and Subjectivity in the Twenty-First Century* (Princeton, N.J.: Princeton University Press, 2007), 10.

48. Human Longevity Inc., "Take Control of Your Health with Health Nucleus," http://www.humanlongevity.com/ (accessed January 23, 2018).

49. Human Longevity Inc.

50. Holstein and Minkler, "Self, Society, and the 'New Gerontology,'" 790, citing Meredith Minkler, "Personal Responsibility for Health? A Review of the Arguments and the Evidence at Century's End," *Health Education and Behavior* 26, no. 1 (1999): 121–40.

51. Katz and Marshall, "Is the Functional 'Normal'?," 64–65.

52. Brett Neilson, "Globalization and the Biopolitics of Aging," *CR: The New Centennial Review* 3, no. 2 (2003): 175.

53. Holstein and Minkler, "Self, Society, and the 'New Gerontology,'" 793. Importantly, the discourse of productive aging and third age intersects with and supports an anti-aging industry and relies on ageist insecurities that marginalize old people in gendered ways—e.g., older bodies that are antifeminine or antimasculine are ostracized and subject to social and medical adjustment.

54. Holstein and Minkler, 793.

55. Holstein and Minkler, 793.

56. Holstein and Minkler, 794.

57. Mykytyn, "Anti-aging Is Not Necessarily Anti-death," 219.

58. Céline Lafontaine, "The Postmortal Condition: From the Biomedical Deconstruction of Death to the Extension of Longevity," *Science as Culture* 18, no. 3 (2009): 309.

59. Neilson, "Globalization and the Biopolitics of Aging," 175.

60. *Biofinancialization* here refers to the metrics used to determine economic policies around health and aging.

61. Emma Whyte Laurie, "Who Lives, Who Dies, Who Cares? Valuing Life through the Disability-Adjusted Life Year Measurement," *Transactions of the Institute of British Geographers* 40, no. 1 (2015): 85.

62. Kaufman, "Making Longevity," 317.

63. Ayo Wahlberg and Nikolas Rose, "The Governmentalization of Living," *Economy and Society* 44, no. 1 (2015): 60–90.

64. Wahlberg and Rose.

65. Katherine E. Kenny, "The Biopolitics of Global Health: Life and Death in Neoliberal Time," *Journal of Sociology* 51, no. 1 (2015): 11.

66. Laurie, "Who Lives, Who Dies, Who Cares?," 82, citing Sudhir Anand and Kara Hanson, "Disability-Adjusted Life Years: A Critical Review," *Journal of Health Economics* 16, no. 6 (1997): 688.

67. Christopher J. L. Murray, Theo Vos, Rafael Lozano, Mohsen Naghavi, Abraham D. Flaxman, Catherine Michaud, Majid Ezzati et al., "Disability-Adjusted Life Years (DALYs) for 291 Diseases and Injuries in 21 Regions, 1990–2010: A Systematic Analysis for the Global Burden of Disease Study 2010," *Lancet* 380, no. 9859 (2012): 2197–2223.

68. Emma Whyte Laurie importantly notes, "They [DALYs] are ostensibly employed to legitimize intervention rather than justify abandonment"; however, "various aspects of the DALY measurement are highly problematic and deeply rooted within a capitalist thinking that considers health in relation to economic productivity." See Laurie, "Who Lives, Who Dies, Who Cares?," 80.

69. Kenny, "Biopolitics of Global Health," 9.

70. Kenny, 16.

71. Laurie, "Who Lives, Who Dies, Who Cares?," 76.

72. David C. Thomasma, "Moving the Aged into the House of the Dead: A Critique of Ageist Social Policy," *Journal of the American Geriatrics Society* 37, no. 2 (1989): 170, cited in Kevin Morgan, *Gerontology: Responding to an Ageing Society* (London: Jessica Kingsley/British Society of Gerontology, 1992), 132.

73. See, e.g., Morgan, *Gerontology.*

74. Henry A. Giroux, "Reading Hurricane Katrina: Race, Class, and the Biopolitics of Disposability," *College Literature* 33, no. 3 (2006): 171–96; Giroux, "Violence, Katrina, and the Biopolitics of Disposability," *Theory, Culture, and Society* 24, no. 7–8 (2007): 305–9.

75. Harris, "QALYfying the Value of Human Life," 108.

76. S. Lochlann Jain, "The Mortality Effect: Counting the Dead in the Cancer Trial," *Public Culture* 22, no. 1 (2010): 89–117.

77. Kelly Fritsch, "Cripping Neoliberal Futurity: Marking the Elsewhere and Elsewhen of Desiring Otherwise," *Feral Feminisms*, no. 5 (2016): 11–26.

78. Sharon R. Kaufman and Lakshmi Fjord, "Medicare, Ethics, and Reflexive Longevity: Governing Time and Treatment in an Aging Society," *Medical Anthropology Quarterly* 25, no. 2 (2011): 1–2.

79. Sharon R. Kaufman, Janet K. Shim, and Ann J. Russ, "Revisiting the Biomedicalization of Aging: Clinical Trends and Ethical Challenges," *Gerontologist* 44, no. 6 (2004): 731.

80. Janet K. Shim, Ann J. Russ, and Sharon R. Kaufman, "Risk, Life Extension and the Pursuit of Medical Possibility," *Sociology of Health and Illness* 28, no. 4 (2006): 485. See also Kaufman and Fjord, "Medicare, Ethics, and Reflexive Longevity"; Sharon R. Kaufman, "Time, Clinic Technologies, and the Making of Reflexive Longevity: The Cultural Work of Time Left in an Ageing Society," *Sociology of Health and Illness* 32, no. 2 (2010): 225–37; and Akse Juul Lassen and Michael Anderson, "What Enhancement Techniques Suggest about the Good Death," *Culture Unbound* 8 (2016): 104–21.

81. Shim et al., "Risk, Life Extension," 486, emphasis added.

82. Kaufman and Fjord, "Medicare, Ethics, and Reflexive Longevity," 2.

83. Kaufman and Fjord, 5.

84. Shim et al., "Risk, Life Extension," 497.

85. On risk discourse, see the late sociologist Ulrich Beck's work, such as *Risk Society: Towards a New Modernity* (London: Sage, 1992). Also François Ewald,

"Insurance and Risk," in *The Foucault Effect: Studies in Governmentality*, ed. Graham Burchell, Colin Gordon, and Peter Miller. 197–210 (Chicago: University of Chicago Press, 1991); Rose, *Politics of Life Itself*, 70–73; Deborah Lupton, *Risk* (London: Routledge, 1999); and Ian Hacking, *The Taming of Chance* (Cambridge: Cambridge University Press, 1990).

86. "An ICD is a battery-powered device placed under the skin that keeps track of your heart rate.... If an abnormal heart rhythm is detected the device will deliver an electric shock to restore a normal heartbeat if your heart is beating chaotically and much too fast." See the American Heart Association, "Implantable Cardioverter Defibrillator (ICD)," http://www.heart.org/HEARTORG/Conditions/Arrhythmia/PreventionTreatmentofArrhythmia/Implantable-Cardioverter-Defibrillator-ICD_UCM_448478_Article.jsp# (accessed December 19, 2017).

87. Shim et al., "Risk, Life Extension"; Steve Phurrough, JoAnna Farrell, and Joseph Chin, "Decision Memorandum for Implantable Cardioverter Defibrillators (ICDs)," CAG-00157N, https://www.cms.gov/medicare-coverage-database/details/nca-decision-memo.aspx?NCAId=39&fromdb=true (accessed December 18, 2017); Richard I. Fogel, Andrew E. Epstein, N. A. Mark Estes III, Bruce D. Lindsay, John P. DiMarco, Mark S. Kremers, Suraj Kapa, Ralph G. Brindis, and Andrea M. Russo, "The Disconnect between the Guidelines, the Appropriate Use Criteria, and Reimbursement Coverage Decisions: The Ultimate Dilemma," *Journal of the American College of Cardiology* 63, no. 1 (2014): 12–14.

88. Medtronic, "Hospital and Physician Reimbursement Guide for ICD Implants," July 2014, http://www.medtronic.com/content/dam/medtronic-com-m/mdt/crdm/documents/july2014-reimburse-guide-icd.pdf (accessed December 18, 2017).

89. Shim et al., "Risk, Life Extension," 490–91.

90. Lassen and Anderson, "What Enhancement Techniques Suggest about the Good Death," 110.

91. Harry Moody, cited in Lassen and Anderson, 110–11; Sara Manning Peskin, "The Symptoms of Protracted Dying," *New York Times*, October 24, 2017, https://www.nytimes.com/2017/10/24/well/live/the-symptoms-of-protracted-dying.html (accessed December 1, 2017).

92. Aimee Swartz, "James Fries: Healthy Aging Pioneer," *American Journal of Public Health* 98, no. 7 (2008): 1163.

93. American Psychological Association, "End-of-Life Care Fact Sheet," http://www.apa.org/pi/aging/programs/eol/end-of-life-factsheet.pdf (accessed December 20, 2017).

94. By 2008, the system was up to its twenty-fifth version, and there were 999 categories (ending with "ungroupable"). See the Centers for Medicare and Medicaid Services (CMS) listing at https://www.cms.gov/Research-Statistics-Data-and-Systems/Statistics-Trends-and-Reports/MedicareFeeforSvcPartsAB

/downloads/DRGdesc08.pdf (accessed December 20, 2017). For the latest DRG categorizations, refer to CMS, "LTC-DRG Files," https://www.cms.gov/Medicare /Medicare-Fee-for-Service-Payment/LongTermCareHospitalPPS/ltcdrg.html (accessed March 8, 2018).

95. Alistair M. Preston, "The Birth of Clinical Accounting: A Study of the Emergence and Transformations of Discourses on Costs and Practices of Accounting in U.S. Hospitals," *Accounting, Organizations, and Society* 17, no. 1 (1992): 92.

96. U.S. House of Representatives, Select Committee on Aging, "Sustaining Quality Health Care under Cost Containment," House Committee Publication 99-499 (Washington, D.C.: Government Printing Office, 1985).

97. Preston also notes that these changes since 1983 have led to "DRG gaming," where hospitals protect their financial interests against the government (vying only for the lucrative DRGs); the heightened economic rationality that is restricting care challenges one of the basic tenets of medicine: to act in the best interest of the patient. Hospitals and doctors now need to juggle this ethic against economic cost control. Preston, "Birth of Clinical Accounting," 95.

98. Bradford H. Gray, ed., *For-Profit Enterprise in Health Care* (Washington, D.C.: National Academies Press, 1986), https://www.ncbi.nlm.nih.gov/books /NBK217906/ (accessed March 8, 2018). For an overview of various dimensions of hospital types, accommodations, and occupancy, see Centers for Disease Control and Prevention (CDC), "Hospitals, Beds, and Occupancy Rates, by Type of Ownership and Size of Hospital: United States, Selected Years 1975–2013," https:// www.cdc.gov/nchs/data/hus/2015/089.pdf (accessed March 8, 2018).

99. Audrey J. Weiss and Anne Elixhauser, "Overview of Hospital Stays in the United States, 2012," Healthcare Cost and Utilization Project Statistical Brief 180, October 2014, https://www.hcup-us.ahrq.gov/reports/statbriefs/sb180-Hospital izations-United-States-2012.pdf (accessed December 17, 2017). For 2016 figures, see Becker's Hospital Review, "60 Things to Know about the Hospital Industry, 2016," January 14, 2016, https://www.beckershospitalreview.com/lists/50-things -to-know-about-the-hospital-industry-2016.html (accessed March 8, 2018).

100. It is also important to note that many hospitals are closing and reopening as ambulatory care centers. This is due to high deductibles, better technology, more case management, and shrinking reimbursement from Medicare and Medicaid. See Melanie Evans, "Hospitals Face Closures as 'a New Day in Healthcare' Dawns," *Modern Healthcare,* February 21, 2015, http://www.modernhealthcare .com/article/20150221/MAGAZINE/302219988 (accessed December 20, 2017). At the same time, many hospitals are expanding into after-hospital care (nursing homes, home care, etc.). In doing so, "hospitals can discharge patients as soon as is medically reasonable, thus minimizing the cost incurred under the hospital DRG, while the patient continues to be revenue-producing in the home care or nursing home setting." Gray, *For-Profit Enterprise in Health Care,* 40.

101. Amal N. Trivedi, Husein Moloo, and Vincent Mor, "Increased Ambulatory Care Copayments and Hospitalizations among the Elderly," *New England Journal of Medicine* 362 (2010): 320–28.

102. This is due to the decline in safety-net hospitals—a category of hospitals that provide a disproportionate level of charity care compared to other facilities. The Patient Protection and Affordable Care Act stipulates that such payments will be reduced over a period of several years. See Becker's Hospital Review, "50 Things to Know about the Hospital Industry."

103. On "social death," refer to Orlando Patterson, *Slavery and Social Death: A Comparative Study* (Cambridge, Mass.: Harvard University Press, 1982).

104. Nancy Ettlinger, "A Relational Approach to an Analytics of Resistance: Towards a Humanity of Care for the Infirm Elderly," *Foucault Studies* 23 (2017): 110.

105. Ettlinger, 111.

106. Ettlinger, 116. Also see CDC, "Nursing Home Care," https://www.cdc.gov/nchs/fastats/nursing-home-care.htm (accessed March 8, 2018).

107. Phillip C. Aka, Lucinda M. Deason, and Augustine Hammond, "Political Factors and the Enforcement of the Nursing Home Regulatory Regime," *Journal of Law and Health* 24, no. 1 (2011): 32.

108. Aka et al., 31.

109. Ettlinger, "A Relational Approach to an Analytics of Resistance," 116.

110. Katie Thomas, "In Race for Medicare Dollars, Nursing Home Care May Lag," *New York Times,* April 14, 2015, https://www.nytimes.com/2015/04/15/business/as-nursing-homes-chase-lucrative-patients-quality-of-care-is-said-to-lag.html (accessed March 8, 2018).

111. U.S. Department of Justice, "Nursing Home Operator to Pay $48 Million to Resolve Allegations That Six California Facilities Billed for Unnecessary Therapy," https://www.justice.gov/opa/pr/nursing-home-operator-pay-48-million-resolve-allegations-six-california-facilities-billed (accessed March 8, 2018).

112. Medford Multicare Center, http://www.medfordmulticare.org/ (accessed December 20, 2017).

113. Thomas, "In Race for Medicare Dollars."

114. Aka et al., "Political Factors," 15. See also Charles Duhigg, "At Many Homes, More Profit and Less Nursing," *New York Times,* September 23, 2007, http://www.nytimes.com/2007/09/23/business/23nursing.html (accessed March 8, 2018).

115. For more on "post-hospital syndrome," see Harlan M. Krumholz, "Post-hospital Syndrome—An Acquired, Transient Condition of Generalized Risk," *New England Journal of Medicine* 368 (2013): 100–102, http://www.nejm.org/doi/full/10.1056/nejmp1212324 (accessed March 8, 2018).

116. Ettlinger, "A Relational Approach to an Analytics of Resistance," 124.

117. Ettlinger, 127.

118. On Obama-era health care reforms related to nursing homes, see Aka et al., "Political Factors," 28. On the Trump administration's rolling back of these initiatives, refer to Jordan Rau, "Trump Administration Eases Nursing Home Fines in Victory for Industry," *New York Times,* December 24, 2017, https:// www.nytimes.com/2017/12/24/business/trump-administration-nursing-home -penalties.html (accessed March 8, 2018).

119. U.S. Government Accountability Office, "Nursing Homes: Federal Moni- toring Surveys Demonstrate Continued Understatement of Serious Care Prob- lems and CMS Oversight Weakness," GAO-08-517, May 2008, https://www.gao .gov/new.items/d08517.pdf (accessed March 8, 2018).

120. See "Nursing Home Quality: CMS Should Continue to Improve Data and Oversight," October 30, 2015, https://www.gao.gov/products/GAO-16-33 (accessed January 20, 2017).

121. National Hospice and Palliative Care Organization, "Facts and Figures: Hospice Care in America," 2017, https://www.nhpco.org/sites/default/files/pub lic/Statistics_Research/2017_Facts_Figures.pdf (accessed April 30, 2019).

122. Norma Jean Dawson, "Need Satisfaction in Terminal Care Settings," *So- cial Science and Medicine* 32, no. 1 (1991): 83–87; Laura Hanson, Marion Danis, and Joanne Garrett, "What Is Wrong with End-of-Life Care? Opinions of Be- reaved Family Members," *Journal of the American Geriatrics Society* 45, no. 11 (1997): 1339–44; Joan M. Teno, B. R. Clarridge, V. Casey, L. C. Welch, T. Wetle, R. Shield, and V. Mor, "Family Perspectives on End-of-Life Care at the Last Place of Care," *Journal of the American Medical Association* 291, no. 1 (2004): 88–93.

123. David J. Casarett and Timothy E. Quill, "'I'm Not Ready for Hospice': Strategies for Timely and Effective Hospice Discussions," *Annals of Internal Medi- cine* 146, no. 6 (2007): 443–49.

124. Stephen R. Connor, Bruce Pyenson, Kathryn Fitch, Carol Spence, and Kosuke Iwasaki, "Comparing Hospice and Nonhospice Patient Survival among Patients Who Die within a Three-Year Window," *Journal of Pain and Symptom Management* 33, no. 3 (2007): 238–46.

125. Julia Lawton, "Contemporary Hospice Care: The Sequestration of the Unbounded Body and 'Dirty Dying,'" *Sociology of Health and Illness* 20, no. 2 (1998): 123.

126. Mark Betancourt, "The Devastating Process of Dying in America without Insurance: What Do People Do When They Can't Afford End-of-Life Care?," *Na- tion,* June 20, 2016, https://www.thenation.com/article/the-devastating-process -of-dying-in-america-without-insurance/ (accessed March 8, 2018). On racial and ethnic disparities in hospice usage, see Lilian Liou Cohen, "Racial/Ethnic Disparities in Hospice Care: A Systematic Review," *Journal of Palliative Medicine* 11, no. 5 (2008): 763–68.

127. Betancourt, "Devastating Process of Dying in America." This growth can

be in part attributed to the rollout of the Medicare Hospice Benefit in 1982, which continued the momentum of hospice care expansion.

128. Refer to the CDC National Center for Health Statistics on hospice care agencies: https://www.cdc.gov/nchs/fastats/hospice-care.htm (accessed March 8, 2018); Joshua E. Perry and Robert C. Stone, "In the Business of Dying: Questioning the Commercialization of Hospice," *Journal of Law, Medicine, and Ethics* 39, no. 2 (2011): 224–34.

129. U.S. Department of Justice, "Chemed Corp. and Vitas Hospice Services Agree to Pay $75 Million to Resolve False Claims Act Allegations," October 30, 2017, https://www.justice.gov/opa/pr/chemed-corp-and-vitas-hospice-services -agree-pay-75-million-resolve-false-claims-act (accessed March 8, 2018).

130. Perry and Stone, "In the Business of Dying," 228.

131. Mykytyn, "Anti-aging Is Not Necessarily Anti-death," 218.

132. Neilson, "Globalization and the Biopolitics of Aging," 179; Matthew Sparke, "Austerity and the Embodiment of Neoliberalism as Ill-Health: Towards a Theory of Biological Sub-citizenship," *Social Science and Medicine* 187 (2017): 287–95.

133. Mykytyn, "Anti-aging Is Not Necessarily Anti-death," 222.

134. John A. Vincent, "Science and Imagery in the 'War on Old Age,'" *Aging and Society* 27, no. 6 (2007): 941–61.

135. Neilson, "Anti-ageing, Cultures, Biopolitics and Globalisation," 160.

136. Kaufman et al., "Revisiting the Biomedicalization of Aging," 731.

137. Cooper, "Resuscitations," 3.

138. AgeLab, http://agelab.mit.edu/agnes-age-gain-now-empathy-system (accessed January 13, 2018).

139. AgeLab.

140. Independent Lens, http://www.pbs.org/independentlens/maggiegrowls /panthers.html (January 13, 2018).

141. Gray Panthers, http://www.graypanthersnyc.org/ (accessed January 13, 2018).

142. The Diverse Elders Coalition (DEC) is supported by five national organizations representing millions of older people throughout the United States: the National Asian Pacific Center on Aging, National Hispanic Council on Aging, National Indian Council on Aging, Sage | Advocacy and Services for LGBT Elders, and Southeast Asia Resource Action Center.

143. Diverse Elders Coalition, https://www.diverseelders.org/ (accessed February 9, 2018).

144. "Diverse Elders Coalition Supports Inclusive Immigration Reform," https://www.diverseelders.org/what-to-know/immigration-reform/ (February 9, 2018).

145. Ann Brenoff, "Why Communes May Be the New Retirement Home,"

Huffington Post, September 10, 2015, https://www.huffingtonpost.com/entry
/communes-may-be-the-new-retirement-home_us_55e47693e4b0b7a963399447
(accessed February 9, 2018).

146. Teresa Mears, "How Baby Boomers Are Creating Their Own Retirement
Communities," *U.S. News,* April 20, 2015, https://money.usnews.com/money
/retirement/articles/2015/04/20/how-baby-boomers-are-creating-their-own
-retirement-communities (accessed February 9, 2018). Cohousing spread in part
due to the book by Kathryn M. Mccamant, Charles Durrett, Ellen Hertzman, and
Charles W. Moore, *Cohousing: A Contemporary Approach to Housing Ourselves*
(1988; repr., Berkeley, Calif.: Ten Speed Press, 1994).

147. Anna Spinner, "Peace, Love, and Social Security: Baby Boomers Retire
to the Commune," *Atlantic,* November 21, 2011, https://www.theatlantic.com
/national/archive/2011/11/peace-love-and-social-security-baby-boomers-retire
-to-the-commune/248583/ (accessed February 9, 2018).

148. Linda Abbit, "Urban Cohousing the Babayaga Way," *Senior Planet,* March
6, 2016, https://seniorplanet.org/senior-housing-alternatives-urban-cohousing
-the-babayaga-way/ (accessed February 10, 2018).

149. Kimberley Fowler, "Shared Housing for Seniors," *Senior Living* (blog), February 27, 2017, https://www.aplaceformom.com/blog/2-27-17-shared-housing
-for-seniors/ (accessed February 10, 2018).

150. Ellen Ryan, "20 Questions and Answers about Cohousing," AARP, January 2016, https://www.aarp.org/livable-communities/housing/info-2016/ques
tions-answers-about-cohousing.html (accessed February 9, 2018); Cohousing
Association of the United States, "Aging in Cohousing," http://www.cohousing
.org/aging (accessed February 10, 2018).

151. Golden Girls Network, https://goldengirlsnetwork.com/ (accessed February 10, 2018).

152. Abbit, "Urban Cohousing the Babayaga Way."

153. Abbit.

154. "Baba Yaga Place—Toronto," http://www.babayagaplace.ca/ (accessed
February 10, 2018).

155. Abbit, "Urban Cohousing the Babayaga Way"; "Baba Yaga Place—Toronto."

156. "The Fellowship Community: An Inter-generational Care Community,"
http://www.fellowshipcommunity.org/ (accessed February 10, 2018).

157. The reasons for multigenerational housing are diverse: the prohibitive
cost of senior care, unemployed family members, young adults in debt and hoping
to save money. According to the Pew Research Center, in 2014, a record 60.6 million people, or 19 percent of the U.S. population, lived with multiple generations
under one roof. Refer to Kavita Daswani, "Multigenerational Homes for Modern Families," *Los Angeles Times,* June 3, 2016, http://www.latimes.com/business
/realestate/hot-property/la-fi-hp-multigenerational-homes-20160604-snap-story

.html (accessed February 10, 2018); Janet Morrissey, "Multigenerational Homes That Fit Just Right," April 8, 2016, https://www.nytimes.com/2016/04/09/your -money/multigenerational-homes-that-fit-just-right.html (accessed February 10, 2018).

158. "Five Core Values of TimeBanking," https://timebanks.org/ (accessed February 10, 2018).

159. Jeff Anderson, "How Time-Banks Promote the Dignity of Seniors," June 14, 2013, https://www.assistedliving.com/time-banks-for-seniors/ (accessed February 10, 2018); Ed Collom, "Engagement of the Elderly in Time Banking: The Potential for Social Capital Generation in an Aging Society," *Journal of Aging and Social Policy* 20, no. 4 (2008): 414–36.

160. Eric TC, "Combining Elderly Care Centers with Preschools: An Idea for Timebanks," July 13, 2015, https://timebanks.org/combining-elderly-care -centers-with-preschools-an-idea-for-timebanks/ (accessed February 10, 2018).

161. "A Time-Banking Scheme Aims to Overcome Britain's Crisis in Care for the Elderly," *Economist,* December 17, 2016, https://www.economist.com/news /britain/21711844-young-people-who-volunteer-now-could-bank-hours-credit -be-redeemed-kind-their-own (accessed February 10, 2018).

162. One of the authors was involved in a project of this kind in Cleveland, Ohio, during college in the 1990s.

163. Generations United, "Shared Sites," https://www.gu.org/what-we-do /public-policy/shared-sites/ (accessed April 30, 2019).

164. Emily DeRuiter, "Adopt-a-Grandparent Is a Co-learning Experience," *Central Michigan Life,* March 31, 2015, http://www.cm-life.com/article/2015/03 /adopt-a-grandparent (accessed February 10, 2018); Ann Brenoff, "Adopt-a-Grandparent Programs Reap Awesome Benefits for Both Sides," *Huffington Post,* April 7, 2015, https://www.huffingtonpost.com/2015/04/07/adopt-a-grandparent -awesome-benefits_n_7012274.html (accessed February 10, 2018).

165. Heather Berlin, "Why We Should Adopt an Elder," *The Forum* (blog), July 5, 2012, http://www.bbc.com/future/story/20120705-why-we-should-adopt-an -elder (accessed February 10, 2018).

166. See Karen Zivi's review of Ben Golder's book *Foucault and the Politics of Rights* (Stanford, Calif.: Stanford University Press, 2015) in *Contemporary Political Theory* 16, no. 2 (2017): 314.

167. Golder, *Foucault and the Politics of Rights.*

168. Golder.

169. Karen Zivi, *Making Rights Claims: A Practice of Democratic Citizenship* (New York: Oxford University Press, 2012), 80.

170. Zivi, quoting Michel Foucault, "The Social Triumph of the Sexual Will," in *Ethics: Subjectivity and Truth,* ed. Paul Rabinow, trans. Robert Hurley et al. (1982; repr., New York: New Press, 1997), 160.

5. Green

1. Deborah Posel and Pamila Gupta, "The Life of the Corpse: Framing Reflections and Questions," *African Studies* 68, no. 3 (2009): 300. Posel and Gupta state, "The regularization of death is inseparable from what Michel Foucault (2003) termed biopolitics" (300).

2. Death studies scholars have explored the complex existence of the corpse: it is a material object that may temporarily circulate but ultimately requires removal/containment. Moreover, dead bodies can anchor social platforms and geographies of power. Refer to Jacque Lynn Foltyn, "The Corpse in Contemporary Culture: Identifying, Transacting, and Recoding the Dead Body in the Twenty-First Century," *Mortality* 13, no. 2 (2008): 99–104; Katherine Verdery, *The Political Lives of Dead Bodies* (New York: Columbia University Press, 1999); Craig Young and Duncan Light, "Corpses, Dead Body Politics and Agency in Human Geography: Following the Corpse of Dr. Petru Groza," *Transactions of the Institute of British Geographers* 38 (2013): 135–48.

3. Philip R. Olson, "Corpses, Technologies, and Cultures," CFP for Open Session 59, Joint Meeting of Society for Social Studies of Science (4S) and Sociedad Latinoamericana de Estudios Sociales de la Ciencia y la Tecnología (ESO-CITE), August 20–23, 2014, Buenos Aires, Argentina, posted on *Discard Studies* (blog), January 24, 2014, http://discardstudies.com/2014/01/24/cfp-corpses-technologies-and-cultures/ (accessed August 5, 2016).

4. Recent death studies scholarship has examined the changing composition of bodies, interactions with land/nature, and technologies of disposal and commemoration. Geographers have also contributed political geographies of dead bodies and research on the importance of space, place, and landscape in the way that death and mourning are imagined and lived, and the differing attitudes toward death related to spaces of dying, grieving, and memorialization. See note 15.

5. *Bioremediation* is a waste management technique that involves the use of organisms to remove or neutralize pollutants from a contaminated site—or, more generally, to remedy something, in particular reversing or stopping environmental damage.

6. We employ the term *biopresence* as inspired by Georg Tremmel and Shiho Fukuhara's project Biopresence: Human DNA Trees, 2007, http://www.biopresence.com/description.html (accessed January 17, 2017).

7. Henry A. Giroux, "Reading Hurricane Katrina: Race, Class, and the Biopolitics of Disposability," *College Literature* 33, no. 3 (2006): 171–96; Giroux, "Violence, Katrina, and the Biopolitics of Disposability," *Theory, Culture, and Society* 24, no. 7–8 (2007): 305–9.

8. Clare Madge, "Living through, Living with and Living on from Breast

Cancer in the UK: Creative Cathartic Methodologies, Cancerous Spaces and a Politics of Compassion," *Social and Cultural Geography* 17, no. 2 (2016): 207–32.

9. Michel Foucault, "17 March 1976," in *Society Must Be Defended: Lectures at the College de France 1975–1976,* ed. Mauro Bertani and Alessandro Fontana, trans. David Macey (New York: Picador, 2003), 254–55.

10. Young and Light, "Corpses, Dead Body Politics."

11. This transition included a shift in the nomenclature and organization of the home: the "parlour" moved outside of the private home (supplanted by the professional funeral parlour) and was renamed the "living room." Death work also shifted from largely informal women's work to the male-dominated funeral profession.

12. Peter Clark and Isabelle Szmigin, "The Structural Captivity of the Funeral Consumer: An Anglo-American Comparison," July 7–9, 2003, Critical Management Studies, Lancaster University, 2, http://www.mngt.waikato.ac.nz/ejrot/cmsconference/2003/proceedings/criticalmarketing/Clark.pdf (accessed January 12, 2017).

13. Young and Light, "Corpses, Dead Body Politics"; Margaret Schwartz, "An Iconography of Flesh: How Corpses Mean as Matter," *Communication +1* 2, no. 1 (2013): 1–16.

14. U.S. Department of the Interior, National Park Service, "National Register Bulletin: Guidelines for Evaluating and Registering Cemeteries and Burial Places," 1992, http://www.nps.gov/nr/publications/bulletins/nrb41/nrb41_5.htm (accessed January 12, 2017).

15. This chapter draws on a rich literature that explores deathscapes and geographies of the dead and dying (much of it in the United Kingdom), e.g., Andy Clayden, Jenny Hockey, and Mark Powell, "Natural Burial: The De-materialising of Death?," in *The Matter of Death: Space, Place and Materiality,* ed. Jenny Hockey, Carol Komaromy, and Kate Woodthorpe, 148–64 (London: Palgrave Macmillan, 2010); Hannah Rumble, John Troyer, Tony Walter, and Kate Woodthorpe, "Disposal or Dispersal? Environmentalism and Final Treatment of the British Dead," *Mortality* 19, no. 3 (2014): 243–60; Richard Yarwood, James D. Sidaway, Claire Kelly, and Susie Stillwell, "Sustainable Deathstyles? The Geography of Green Burials in Britain," *Geographical Journal* 181, no. 2 (2015): 172–84; Jenny Hockey, Trish Green, Andy Clayden, and Mark Powell, "Landscapes of the Dead? Natural Burial and the Materialization of Absence," *Journal of Material Culture* 17, no. 2 (2012): 115–32; Olivia Stevenson, Charlotte Kenten, and Avril Maddrell, "And Now the End Is Near: Enlivening and Politicising the Geographies of Dying, Death and Mourning," *Social and Cultural Geography* 17, no. 2 (2016): 153–65; and Avril Maddrell, "Mapping Grief: A Conceptual Framework for Understanding the Spatial Dimensions of Bereavement, Mourning and Remembrance," *Social and Cultural Geography* 17, no. 2 (2016): 166–88. See also Jean-Robert Pitte, "A Short Cultural Geography of Death and the Dead," *GeoJournal* 60, no. 4 (2004):

345–51; Tan Boon Hui and Brenda S. A. Yeoh, "The 'Remains of the Dead': Spatial Politics of Nation-Building in Post-War Singapore," *Human Ecology Review* 9, no. 1 (2002): 1–13; and Lily Kong, "Cemeteries, Columbaria, Memorials and Mausoleums: Narrative and Interpretation in the Study of Deathscapes in Geography," *Australian Geographical Studies* 37, no. 1 (1999): 1–10.

16. Doris Francis, "Cemeteries as Cultural Landscapes," *Mortality* 8, no. 2 (2003): 224; Suzanne Kelly, "Dead Bodies That Matter: Toward a New Ecology of Human Death in American Culture," *Journal of American Culture* 35, no. 1 (2012): 37–51; Julie Rugg, "Lawn Cemeteries: The Emergence of a New Landscape of Death," *Urban History* 33, no. 2 (2006): 213–33.

17. Because of space limitations, we are unable to incorporate cemetery reforms, from the rural cemetery movement to "modern" cemetery planning and the City Beautiful memorial park.

18. Yarwood et al., "Sustainable Deathstyles?," 174; Hockey et al., "Landscapes of the Dead?," 124.

19. Alexandra Harker, "Landscapes of the Dead: An Argument for Conservation Burial," *Berkeley Planning Journal* 25, no. 1 (2012): 150–59; Funeral Consumers Alliance, "Green Burial," November 26, 2007, https://funerals.org /greenburial/ (accessed January 17, 2018).

20. Bruna Oliveira, Paula Quinteiro, Carla Caetano, Helena Nadais, Luís Arroja, Eduardo Ferreira da Silva, and Manuel Senos Matias, "Burial Grounds' Impact on Groundwater and Public Health: An Overview," *Water and Environment Journal* 27 (2013): 99–106; Johnny P. Stowe Jr., Elise Vernon Schmidt, and Deborah Green, "Toxic Burials: The Final Insult," *Conservation Biology* 15, no. 6 (2001): 1817–19; Józef Żychowski, "Impact of Cemeteries on Groundwater Chemistry: A Review," *Catena* 93 (2012): 29–37.

21. Kelly, "Dead Bodies That Matter." See also Elizabeth J. Emerick, "Death and the Corpse: An Analysis of the Treatment of Death and Dead Bodies in Contemporary American Society," *Anthropology of Consciousness* 11, no. 1–2 (2000): 34–48.

22. National Funeral Directors Association, http://www.nfda.org/news /media-center/nfda-news-releases/id/1310/2016-nfda-cremation-and-burial -report-released-rate-of-cremation-surpasses-that-of-burial-in-2015 (accessed January 17, 2017).

23. Yarwood et al., "Sustainable Deathstyles?," 174. This includes concerns over the "turnover" of interred bodies: unless high maintenance costs are paid, cemeteries will typically remove coffins after twenty years and rebury bodies in common graves. As a result, cremation with smaller plots for urns, not coffins, is growing.

24. For data on cremation toxicity, consult Montse Mari and José L. Domingo, "Toxic Emissions from Crematories: A Review," *Environment International* 36 (2010): 131–37; Louise Canning and Isabelle Szmigin, "Death and Disposal:

The Universal, Environmental Dilemma," *Journal of Marketing Management* 26, no. 11–12 (2010): 1129–42.

25. Karen Sprey, "Resomation and Corpse-Composting: Alternatives to Cremation and Burial," *New Atlas,* July 5, 2010, http://newatlas.com/resomation-corpse-composting-green-burial/15603/ (accessed January 15, 2017).

26. For discussion of the broad social arenas and markets of "sustainability," refer to Adrian Parr, *Hijacking Sustainability* (Cambridge, Mass.: MIT Press, 2009); Parr, *The Wrath of Capital: Neoliberalism and Climate Change Politics* (New York: Columbia University Press, 2012).

27. Rumble et al., "Disposal or Dispersal?"

28. "Exploitation" of the corpse is not necessarily negative—the phrase here merely emphasizes the application of the dead body/parts to other uses.

29. Foltyn, "Corpse in Contemporary Culture," 200.

30. Catherine Waldby, *The Visible Human Project: Informatic Bodies and Posthuman Medicine* (London: Routledge, 2000); see also Stefan Helmreich, "Species of Biocapital," *Science as Culture* 17, no. 4 (2008): 463–78.

31. Margaret Lock on the reinvention of "death" for U.S. organ transplantation/donation: *Twice Dead: Organ Transplants and the Reinvention of Death* (Berkeley: University of California Press, 2002).

32. U.S. Department of Health and Human Services/Organdonor.gov, "Registration Statistics," https://www.organdonor.gov/statistics-stories/statistics.html (accessed May 6, 2019).

33. Donate Life America, https://www.donatelife.net/statistics/ (accessed January 17, 2017).

34. BioGift, http://www.biogift.org/ (accessed January 17, 2017).

35. Mayo Clinic, http://www.mayoclinic.org/body-donation/overview (accessed January 17, 2017).

36. *Taphonomy* is the study of decaying organisms. Monica Raymunt, "Down on the Body Farm: Inside the Dirty World of Forensic Science," *Atlantic,* December 2, 2010, http://www.theatlantic.com/technology/archive/2010/12/down-on-the-body-farm-inside-the-dirty-world-of-forensic-science/67241/ (accessed August 5, 2016); Robert Gannon, "The Body Farm," *Popular Science* 251, no. 3 (1997): 77.

37. Forensic Anthropology Center, https://fac.utk.edu/ (accessed January 17, 2017).

38. Donna Haraway, *Simians, Cyborgs, and Women: The Reinvention of Nature* (New York: Routledge, 1991).

39. This process is increasingly regulated by state guidelines on disposing and recycling crematory metals. The laws are aimed at resolving legal uncertainties about who owns the right to the salvaged material.

40. Implant Recycling, http://www.implantrecycling.com/home.html (accessed January 15, 2017).

41. Sandy Bauers, "Ultimate Recycling: Artificial Joints after Recycling," *Inquirer,* February 24, 2012, https://www.philly.com/philly/news/homepage/2012 0224_Ultimate_recycling__Artificial_joints_after_cremation.html (accessed January 13, 2017).

42. Dr. John Troyer, Deputy Director of the Centre for Death and Society at the University of Bath, quoted in Andrew Mourant, "Should the Excess Heat from Cremation Be Recycled?," *The Guardian,* April 25, 2011, http://www.theguardian .com/education/2011/apr/25/cremation-excess-heat-research (accessed January 13, 2017).

43. Georgina Cooper, "Crematorium May Use Its Heat to Warm Mourners," Reuters, January 9, 2008, http://www.reuters.com/article/2008/01/09/us-britain -cremation-idUSL0925836220080109 (accessed January 13, 2017); *Economist,* "Body Heat," August 6, 2009, http://www.economist.com/node/14191268 (accessed January 13, 2017).

44. Warren McLaren, "Dead People Are Cool: Crematorium Heat Powers Air Conditioning," *Treehugger* (blog), October 8, 2009, http://www.treehugger .com/renewable-energy/dead-people-are-cool-crematorium-heat-powers-air -conditioning.html (accessed January 17, 2017); *Green Futures Magazine,* "Circle of Life: Waste Heat Harnessed from Cremation," July 25, 2011, https://www .forumforthefuture.org/greenfutures/articles/circle-life-waste-heat-harnessed -cremation (accessed January 17, 2017).

45. Justin Nobel, "New Life for Crematories' Heat Waste," *Pacific Standard Magazine,* May 24, 2011, http://www.psmag.com/nature-and-technology/new -life-for-crematories-waste-heat-31501 (accessed January 17, 2017).

46. Virginia Hughes, "Waste Heat Is Free Energy. So Why Aren't We Using It?," *Popular Science,* March 13, 2014, http://www.popsci.com/article/science /waste-heat-free-energy-so-why-arent-we-using-it (accessed January 13, 2017).

47. National Funeral Directors Association, "Statistics," July 30, 2015, http:// nfda.org/media-center/statistics.html (accessed July 8, 2016).

48. Philip R. Olson, "Flush and Bone: Funeralizing Alkaline Hydrolysis in the United States," *Science, Technology, and Human Values* 39, no. 5 (2014): 671.

49. Mayo Clinic, "Body Donation at Mayo Clinic," http://www.mayoclinic .org/body-donation/making-donation (accessed January 13, 2017).

50. C. DeArmond, "Site Visit: Green Cremation, St. Petersburg Funeral Home Offers a Green Way to Go with World's First Commercial Resomator," *2nd Green Revolution* (blog), September 14, 2011, http://2ndgreenrevolution .com/2011/09/14/site-visit-green-cremation-st-petersburg-funeral-home-offers -a-green-way-to-go-with-world's-first-commercial-resomator/ (accessed July 8, 2016). Water accounts for approximately 95 percent of the total solution.

51. U.S. Funerals Online, "Aquamation or Resomation," April 22, 2014, http:// www.us-funerals.com/funeral-articles/aquamation-or-resomation-a-green-alter native-to-the-traditional-funeral.html (accessed January 13, 2017).

52. As of 2018, states that have approved resomation include Colorado, Florida, Georgia, Idaho, Illinois, Kansas, Maine, Maryland, Michigan, Minnesota, Nevada, Oregon, Vermont, and Wyoming. States with pending approval encompass California, New Jersey, New York, North Carolina, Ohio, and Pennsylvania. For analysis of the controversial deployment of alkaline hydrolysis in the United States, see Olson, "Flush and Bone." Resomation Limited started in Scotland; the process was adapted for funeral home use by the Mayo Clinic in its anatomy bequest program (since 2007). The first resomation machine was installed in the Anderson-McQueen Funeral Home in St. Petersburg, Florida, followed by the Bradshaw Celebration of Life Center in Stillwater, Minnesota. Another alternative funeral method, "cryomation" or "promession," lowers emissions without extensive water use; for more detail, refer to Promessa, "Ecological Burial," 2014, http://www.promessa.se/ (accessed January 17, 2017).

53. Rumble et al., "Disposal or Dispersal?," 248: "The fuel for burning a human body comes only in part from the gas burners and from the wood of the coffin; it also comes substantially from the body's own fat. Thus, recycling the heat produced in cremation entails burning the dead's fat to warm the living."

54. Kelly, "Dead Bodies That Matter," 48.

55. Sarah Bezan, "Necro-Eco: The Ecology of Death in Jim Crace's *Being Dead*," *Mosaic* 48, no. 3 (2015): 191–207.

56. This is a play on the words "cradle to cradle," a trademarked design concept by William McDonough and Michael Braungart. See the documentary film *Waste=Food,* dir. Rob van Hattum, 2006 (51 min.). The idea that the human body and human decomposition could be reconceived as "food" for nature or animals is also explored by environmental activist-writers: Edward Abbey, *Desert Solitaire* (New York: Ballantine Books, 1985); Val Plumwood, "Prey to a Crocodile," *Aisling Magazine* 30 (2002), http://www.aislingmagazine.com/aislingmagazine/articles/TAM30/ValPlumwood.html (accessed May 3, 2019).

57. Urban Death Project, http://urbandeathproject.org/#overview (accessed January 15, 2017).

58. Urban Death Project.

59. Jae Rhim Lee, "My Mushroom Burial Suit," TEDGlobal 2011, https://www.ted.com/talks/jae_rhim_lee?language=en (accessed January 17, 2017); Coeio, "Infinity Burial Suit," http://coeio.com/infinity-burial-suit-2/ (accessed January 17, 2017).

60. Sara J. Marsden, "Green Burial Sites in the United States," U.S. Funerals Online, July 19, 2016, http://www.us-funerals.com/funeral-articles/directory-of-green-burial-sites-in-the-united-states.html (accessed January 15, 2018).

61. Green Burial Council, https://www.greenburialcouncil.org/our_standards.html (accessed May 3, 2019).

62. The most advanced Three-Leaf ranking is reserved for conservation burial grounds that must protect an area of land specifically designated for conserva-

tion, i.e., a conservation easement or deed restriction guaranteeing long-term stewardship.

63. This median figure does not include cemetery vault, monument/marker, fees for opening/closing the plot, crematory fee (if selected), or items like flowers, burial clothing, an obituary, or clergy fees. If a conservation cemetery is chosen, perpetual care costs are less than a traditional cemetery: the money is applied toward maintaining trails rather than lawn mowing and fighting invasive plant species. A plant or engraved boulder can be used to mark the grave—or nothing but knowledge of the GPS coordinates.

64. Kelly, "Dead Bodies That Matter," 50. In most states, it is legal to care for your own dead; however, this is heavily conditioned—if not wholly prohibited—by law at other scales, particularly municipal regulations. For more information, refer to Funerals Online, "What Do I Do If I Can't Afford a Funeral?," June 8, 2013, http://www.us-funerals.com/funeral-articles/what-to-do-if-i-cannot-afford-a -funeral.html (accessed January 13, 2017). A growing number of "death mid-wives" and "home death guides" help people navigate "act local" death options. The National Home Funeral Alliance coordinates a code of ethics and rules to govern home death advisors. Other efforts focus on advanced planning resources and education about death care.

65. Eternity Cardboard Casket, http://www.eeternity.com/ (accessed January 17, 2017).

66. Kinkaraco, http://kinkaraco.com/pages/history (accessed January 17, 2017).

67. ARKA Acorn Urn, http://funerals.naturalburialcompany.com/products /ARKA-Acorn-Urn-%252d-Green.html (accessed January 17, 2017); Bios Urn, https://urnabios.com/ (accessed January 17, 2017); Shell Urn, https://www.pas sagesinternational.com/biodegradable-urns/water/shell-urns/ (accessed May 3, 2019).

68. LifeGem, http://www.lifegem.com/images/LifeGem_Web_Brochure_Cur rent.pdf (accessed January 17, 2017). The first U.S. company to extract carbon from human remains, LifeGem provides unique identifiers and etching options and guarantees certification of the diamond by authorized gemologists. Depend-ing on weight, color, and carats, the price ranges from $2,690 to $24,999.

69. Marisa Kakoulas, "Cremation Ashes Memorial Tattoo," May 9, 2011, http://www.needlesandsins.com/2011/05/cremation-ashes-memorial-tattoo.html (accessed January 17, 2017).

70. Eternal Reefs, "What Is an Eternal Reef?," 2014, http://eternalreefs.com /the-eternal-reefs-story/what-is-an-eternal-reef/ (accessed January 17, 2017).

71. Eternal Reefs, http://eternalreefs.com/ (accessed January 17, 2017).

72. Biopresence, "Biopresence. Human DNA Trees," 2007, http://www.bio presence.com/description.html (accessed January 17, 2017).

73. Georg Tremmel and Shiho Fukuhara, "Biopresence," http://www.trembl

.org/alumni/01-03/transplant.html (accessed January 17, 2017). Joe Davies is known for his efforts to place fifty thousand of the most popular Wikipedia pages into the DNA of an apple tree to generate a Tree of Knowledge.

74. Natalia Lizama, "Afterlife, but Not as We Know It: Medicine, Technology and the Body Resurrected" (PhD diss., University of Western Australia, Perth, 2008).

75. Foucault, "17 March 1976," 254–55.

76. Achille Mbembe, "Necropolitics," *Public Culture* 15, no. 1 (2003): 11–40; Judith Butler, *Frames of War: When Is Life Grievable?* (New York: Verso, 2010).

77. Posel and Gupta, "Life of the Corpse," 303.

78. A notable exception is the social networking of organ donation charity, such as organ donation circles.

79. *Social death* refers to the "dispossessed" social ontology of the living who are cut off from social ties and suffer the condition of not being accepted as fully human. Prime examples are slavery, apartheid, and racial, gendered, and sexual exclusions and terrorisms. This important theorization extends from Orlando Patterson's work on slavery as one of the most extreme forms of domination. See Orlando Patterson, *Slavery and Social Death: A Comparative Study* (Cambridge, Mass.: Harvard University Press, 1982). For our purposes here, we use the term *social death of death* to explore the privatizing of death as a social relation with the material dead body.

80. The corpse can be said to have a dynamic digital afterlife and online postmortal intersubjectivity/agency; refer to Adam Tucker, "Virtually Dead: The Extension of Social Agency to Corpses and the Dead on Facebook" (honors thesis 53, College of St. Benedict and St. John's University, St. Joseph, Minn., 2014), http://digitalcommons.csbsju.edu/honors_theses/53 (accessed January 17, 2017); Natalie Pennington, "You Don't De-friend the Dead: An Analysis of Grief Communication by College Students through Facebook Profiles," *Death Studies* 37, no. 7 (2013): 617–35; Patrick Stokes, "Ghosts in the Machine: Do the Dead Live on in Facebook?," *Philosophy and Technology* 25, no. 3 (2012): 363–79; Sheila Harper, "The Social Agency of Dead Bodies," *Mortality* 15, no. 4 (2010): 308–22.

81. Olson, "Flush and Bone"; Clark and Szmigin, "Structural Captivity of the Funeral Consumer," 5; Jessica Mitford, "The Undertaker's Racket," *Atlantic Monthly,* June 1963, http://www.theatlantic.com/magazine/archive/1963/06/the-undertakers-racket/305318/ (accessed January 17, 2017).

82. For example, "direct cremation" is now a standard package that includes taking the body to a crematory, placing it in a cardboard container, cremating the body, completing necessary documents, and shipping ashes to the family for keeping or burial/placement in a cemetery. David E. Harrington, "Markets: Preserving Funeral Markets with Ready-to-Embalm Laws," *Journal of Economic Perspectives* 21, no. 4 (2007): 201–16.

83. On the dispossession of human remains via science, anthropology, and museums, refer to Kim TallBear, *Native American DNA: Tribal Belonging and the False Promise of Genetic Science* (Minneapolis: University of Minnesota Press, 2013); Jenny Reardon and Kim TallBear, "'Your DNA Is Our History': Genomics, Anthropology, and the Construction of Whiteness as Property," *Current Anthropology* 53 (2012): S233–45.

84. Harriet A. Washington, *Medical Apartheid: The Dark History of Medical Experimentation on Black Americans from Colonial Times to the Present* (New York: Anchor, 2008); Alondra Nelson, *Body and Soul: The Black Panther Party and the Fight Against Medical Discrimination* (Minneapolis: University of Minnesota Press, 2011); Jenna M. Loyd, *Health Rights Are Civil Rights: Peace and Justice Activism in Los Angeles, 1963–1978* (Minneapolis: University of Minnesota Press, 2014). Also see chapter 2 of this volume.

85. Refer to Nancy Scheper-Hughes, "The Ends of the Body: Commodity Fetishism and the Global Traffic in Organs," *SAIS Review* 22, no. 1 (2002): 61–80.

86. In the United States, organ donation is regulated under the National Organ Transplant Act, a 1984 law that categorizes human organs as a national resource and prohibits their sale. However, there are numerous cases of violation. Refer to David E. Harrington and Edward A. Sayre, "Paying for Bodies, but Not for Organs," *Regulation,* Winter 2006–7, 14–19.

87. Another cost–benefit default of many U.S. states is to utilize prisoners for cemetery labor, at no cost and little concern for any toxic exposure. The category "unknowns" refers to those dead bodies that were not found to be connected—owned—by anyone living, in other words, those unclaimed bodies that therefore became property of the state for disposal. *Potter's field*—a biblical expression referencing a field that was useless to agriculture and could be utilized for the extraction of potter's clay and as a burial site—also known as a common grave, usually refers to a place for the burial of indigent and/or unknown people.

88. For discussion of disappearing bodies, refer to Monica J. Casper and Lisa Jean Moore, *Missing Bodies: The Politics of Visibility* (New York: New York University Press, 2009). For an overview of the controversy over the official U.S. death toll of Puerto Rico, see Alexis R. Santos-Lozada, "Why Puerto Rico's Death Toll from Hurricane Maria Is So Much Higher than Officials Thought," *Conversation,* January 3, 2018, https://theconversation.com/why-puerto-ricos-death-toll-from-hurricane-maria-is-so-much-higher-than-officials-thought-89349 (accessed February 3, 2018).

89. Karla Zabludovsky, "In Texas, a Surge of Migrants Also Means a Surge of Dead Bodies," *Newsweek,* July 24, 2014, http://www.newsweek.com/texas-migrant-country-medical-examiner-busy-260979 (accessed April 15, 2017).

90. Merrit Kennedy, "Lead-Laced Water in Flint: A Step-by-Step Look at the Makings of a Crisis," *Two-Way,* NPR, April 20, 2016, https://www.npr.org

/sections/thetwo-way/2016/04/20/465545378/lead-laced-water-in-flint-a-step
-by-step-look-at-the-makings-of-a-crisis (accessed February 3, 2018); Oona
Goodin-Smith, "Lead in Flint Water Increased Fetal Deaths, Lowered Fertility,
Study Says," *MLive,* October 13, 2017, http://www.mlive.com/news/flint/index
.ssf/2017/09/lead_in_flint_water_increased.html (accessed February 3, 2018);
Keith Matheny, "Study: Flint Water Killed Unborn Babies; Many Moms Who
Drank It Didn't Get Pregnant," September 20, 2017, https://www.freep.com/story
/news/local/michigan/flint-water-crisis/2017/09/20/flint-water-crisis-pregnan
cies/686138001/ (accessed February 3, 2018). For analysis of Flint with respect
to environmental racism and racial capitalism/racial liberalism, refer to Laura
Pulido, "Flint, Environmental Racism, and Racial Capitalism," *Capitalism Nature
Socialism* 27, no. 3 (2016): 1–16; Malini Ranganathan, "Thinking with Flint: Ra-
cial Liberalism and the Roots of an American Water Tragedy," *Capitalism Nature
Socialism* 27, no. 3 (2016): 17–33; Julie Sze, *Environmental Justice in a Moment of
Danger* (Berkeley: University of California Press, forthcoming).

91. Rugg, "Lawn Cemeteries"; Francis, "Cemeteries as Cultural Landscapes."

92. Kelly, "Dead Bodies That Matter," 38.

93. Ellen Stroud, "Dead Bodies in Harlem: Environmental History and the
Geography of Death," in *The Nature of Cities: Culture, Landscape and Urban
Space,* ed. Andrew Isenberg, 62–76 (Rochester, N.Y.: University of Rochester
Press, 2006).

94. David Charles Sloane, *The Last Great Necessity: Cemeteries in American
History* (Baltimore: The Johns Hopkins University Press, 1991).

95. Adonnica Toler, Historian/Museum Assistant at the Ritz Theatre and
Museum in Jacksonville, Florida, quoted in Jacob Long, "Death and Burials: The
Final Frontier for Segregation," *First Coast News,* April 30, 2014, http://www.first
coastnews.com/story/news/local/2014/04/30/segregation-jacksonville-cemetery
-death-burials/8510995/ (accessed July 8, 2016). Ethnic differences, class, age,
family conflicts over birth and marriage, and "strains between communal values
and the autonomy of the socially mobile individual are marked by permanent
mortuary symbols." Refer to Francis, "Cemeteries as Cultural Landscapes," 223.

96. Douglas James Davies, *A Brief History of Death* (Oxford: Blackwell, 1995).

97. This idea draws on Joseph Pugliese's concept of "necrological whiteness,"
which he deploys to explore how "whiteness exercises its signifying grip beyond
the biological life of the subject. . . . The phase of biological death must be seen as
firmly situated within the racializing continuum maintained and reproduced by a
cluster of different institutions, authorities and regulative regimes." See Pugliese,
"Necrological Whiteness: The Racial Prosthetics of Template Bodies," *Continuum*
19, no. 3 (2005): 349.

98. Tony Platt, "UC and Native Americans: Unsettled Remains," *Los Angeles
Times,* June 18, 2013, http://articles.latimes.com/2013/jun/18/opinion/la-oe-platt

-native-american-indian-remains-20130618 (accessed January 15, 2017); *USA Today,* "Black History Dies in Neglected Southern Cemeteries," January 30, 2013, http://www.usatoday.com/story/news/nation/2013/01/30/black-history-dies-in -southern-cemeteries/1877687/ (accessed January 15, 2017). In essentially one month's time in early 2017, three Jewish cemeteries were serially defiled in St. Louis, Philadelphia, and Rochester, along with anti-Semitic threats of violence against Jewish community centers. This has only escalated through 2018 and 2019.

99. The Pensacola Area Cemetery Team (PACT) is a prominent example. Refer to Joe Vinson, "A Community 'PACT' to Preserve, Share Historic Black Cemeteries," Studer Community Institute, March 26, 2015, http://studeri.org /2015/03/a-community-pact-to-preserve-share-historic-black-cemeteries/ (accessed January 15, 2017).

100. For example, Louisville, Kentucky's, St. Joseph of Arimathea Society sends volunteer high school students to serve as pallbearers and handle any religious readings. See Trinity High School's Joseph of Arimathea Society, http://www .trinityrocks.com/students/student-life/clubs-activities/special-interest/joseph -of-arimathea-society/ (September 15, 2017).

101. Congressional Cemetery in Washington, D.C., leads tours of LGBTQ activism that include Leonard Matlovich's tombstone. For examples of historic civil rights actions and funerals, and the crucial infrastructure of black funeral homes for African American community organizing, see Suzanne E. Smith, *To Serve the Living: Funeral Directors and the African American Way of Death* (Cambridge, Mass.: Belknap Press of Harvard University Press, 2010).

102. Stuart Murray, "Thanatopolitics: Reading in Agamben a Rejoinder to Biopolitical Life," *Communication and Critical/Cultural Studies* 5, no. 2 (2008): 203–7.

103. Dave Brennan, "Dying Destitute in the United States," *Funeral Law* (blog), April 2, 2014, http://funerallaw.typepad.com/blog/2014/04/dying-destitute-in -the-united-states.html (accessed July 8, 2016).

Coda

1. Stuart Murray, "Thanatopolitics: On the Use of Death for Mobilizing Political Life," *Polygraph* 18 (2006): 193.

2. Didier Fassin, "Another Politics of Life Is Possible," *Theory, Culture, and Society* 26, no. 5 (2009): 53.

3. Fassin, 57.

4. For an examination of endurance, see Elizabeth Povinelli, *Economies of Abandonment: Social Belonging and Endurance in Late Liberalism* (Durham, S.C.: Duke University Press, 2011), and Povinelli, "The Will to Be Otherwise/The Effort of Endurance," *South Atlantic Quarterly* 111, no. 3 (2012): 453–75.

5. Jacques Derrida, *The Last Interview* (New York: Studio Visit, 2004). In this understanding, survival is "the affirmation of someone who prefers living, and therefore surviving, to death." Note that this is a radically different notion of survival to the one we discuss in chapter 1. There we talk of the survivor narrative, which is predicated on relentless life, optimism, and triumphalism.

6. Didier Fassin, "Ethics of Survival: A Democratic Approach to the Politics of Life," *Humanity: An International Journal of Human Rights, Humanitarianism, and Development* 1, no. 1 (2010): 83.

7. Fassin, 94

8. Murray, "Thanatopolitics," 211.

9. S. Lochlann Jain, "Living in Prognosis: Toward an Elegiac Politics," *Representations* 98 (2007): 90.

10. Peter James Hudson, "The Geographies of Blackness and Anti-Blackness: An Interview with Katherine McKittrick," *CLR James Journal* 20, no. 1–2 (2014): 237. There is obviously a long history and rich present of such activity within black communities.

11. McKittrick brilliantly asserts, "So, for me, one way to dislodge this kind of analytic thinking is to both expose its naturalness (of course violence is wrong and unjust, but why is naming it *naturally* at the heart of our academic *conclusions*!), to draw attention to black thinkers that provide deliberate commentary on the ways in which blackness works against the violence that defines it (so here I look to the work of [Sylvia] Wynter among many many others, Audre Lorde, [Frantz] Fanon, Saidiya Hartman, as well as a whole range of black creative thinkers and musicians), and to demand that this deliberate commentary be central to how we think about and organize the planet and our futures." Hudson, 240.

12. Michel Foucault, "Questions of Method," in *The Foucault Effect: Studies in Governmentality,* ed. Graham Burchell, Colin Gordon, and Peter Miller (Chicago: University of Chicago Press, 1991), 84. Key to Foucault's method is the "immense and proliferating criticizability of things, institutions, practices, and discourses." Refer to Michel Foucault, *Society Must Be Defended: Lectures at the Collège de France 1975–1976,* ed. Mauro Bertani and Alessandro Fontana, trans. David Macey (New York: Picador, 2003), 6.

13. Michel Foucault, "What Is Critique?," in *The Politics of Truth,* ed. Sylvère Lotringer, trans. Lysa Hochroth and Catherine Porter (New York: Semiotext(e), 1997), 45.

14. Again, we take a Foucauldian approach to the question of ethics. Ethics are not morals, in Foucault's formulation. Rather, ethical activity "has to do with actions and choices"; refer to Ladelle McWhorter, *Bodies and Pleasures: Foucault and the Politics of Sexual Normalization* (Bloomington: Indiana University Press, 1999), 195. Also see Foucault's discussion about meditating on death as a form of care in *The Hermeneutics of the Subject: Lectures at the Collège de France, 1981–*

1982 (New York: Palgrave Macmillan, 2005), 355–70. Our understanding of care stems from a feminist ethics of care standpoint. See specifically María Puig de la Bellacasa, "Matters of Care in Technoscience: Assembling Neglected Things," *Social Studies of Science* 41, no. 1 (2011): 85–106, and Joan Tronto, *Moral Boundaries: A Political Argument for an Ethic of Care* (New York: Routledge, 1993).

15. Stuart Murray, "Affirming the Human? The Question of Biopolitics," *Law, Culture, and the Humanities* 12, no. 3 (2016): 495.

16. Vulnerability has been politicized in the theoretical arena and seen as the site from which a potential ethics might emerge. This has been particularly evident in the fields of disability studies, environmental studies, and material feminisms. Studies of biomedicine and bioethics have taken a renewed interest in the theorization of vulnerability and its accompanying ethics. See, for instance, the special issue on "Vulnerability" of the *International Journal of Feminist Approaches to Bioethics* 5, no. 2 (2012).

Index

Page numbers in italics refer to figures.

Nadine Ehlers teaches sociology at the University of Sydney. Her research broadly focuses on the sociocultural study of the body, law, and biomedicine to examine racial and gendered governance. She is author of *Racial Imperatives: Discipline, Performativity, and Struggles against Subjection* and coeditor of *Subprime Health: Debt and Race in U.S. Medicine* (Minnesota, 2017).

Shiloh Krupar is a geographer and Provost's Distinguished Associate Professor at Georgetown University, where she chairs the Culture and Politics program in the School of Foreign Service. Her research explores militarism and nuclear natures, urban cultural politics in China, environmental and financial disasters, and medical geographies of waste. She is author of *Hot Spotter's Report: Military Fables of Toxic Waste* (Minnesota, 2013).